MEDICAL LIMERICKS V

by

William J. Stone, MD

MEDICAL LIMERICKS V

ISBN-13: 978-1517511166
ISBN-10: 151751116X

Library of Congress Control Number 2013905988
CreateSpace, North Charleston, S.C., USA

*Booklet cover, design and all prepress by Mary Margaret
Alsobrook Peel. Ms. Peel is a Medical Illustrator and
currently serves as the Chief of Medical Media at the
Department of Veterans Affairs Medical Center where
she directs illustration, graphic design, photography, and
other visual support for medical, patient and staff teaching
programs.*

Dedicated to
The Faculty of the Department of Medicine
Vanderbilt University School of Medicine

UNUSUAL CELLULITIS

A "man's man", he'd been a Kentucky hoopster.

Swollen red legs; cultures bland, where to refer?

Skin biopsy showed AFB.

Then we got more history.

He was a steady pedicure customer.

Note: Pedicure has been implicated in causing hepatitis B and C, prosthetic valve endocarditis, Herpes simplex, fungal infections, prosthetic knee infections, and non-tuberculous mycobacterial (AFB) furunculosis of the legs. Typically, these AFB are "rapid growers", such as M. fortuitum, M. chelonae, and M. abscessus. Improper maintenance of the whirlpool foot baths is responsible. In this patient a second skin biopsy grew M. chelonae. He was improving on appropriate antimicrobials.

Refs.: NEJM 2002; 346:1366-71; Emerg Infect Dis 2005; 11: 616-618.

FACIAL CELLULITIS

Within a day of dental extraction

He developed a curious reaction.

Facial rash and sores widely,

But with acyclovir IV

He healed to our satisfaction.

Note: This 64 year old man went in for a routine tooth extraction, noted that there was a new hygienist, and became ill on the next evening. He had oral and facial vesicles/ulcers along with a cellulitis on both cheeks. There was no history of herpes, but HSV-1 was identified on DFA. He responded slowly to IV acyclovir. Tests for HIV and HSV-2 were negative. Could the procedure have transmitted HSV-1 that rapidly? HSV-1/2 IgM was (+) at 30.9 (normal 0-0.9). HSV-1/2 IgG was not sent. A literature search for a dental procedure transmitting HSV-1 was negative. However, oral surgery can activate shedding of HSV-1 by any patient, who is an asymptomatic carrier.

Ref. : Oral Dis 2007; 13:414-418.

THE PICTURE OF HEALTH

Claimed hemoptysis, homeless, HIV,

Multiple nodes seen upon a CT.

To HAART he was not adhering.

Cultures showed fungi appearing.

He's doing well on azole therapy.

Note: The house staff admitting him wanted to know
why he was hospitalized, since he looked so well.
The CT had already been done in the ED. Due to the
adenopathy, he received blood and CSF cultures to
rule out an infectious cause. Both grew cryptococci.
Cryptococcal antigen was 1:4 in the CSF (there were
only 10 WBC) and 1:256 in blood. Incidentally, the
hemoptysis was feigned.

Ref.: Clin Infect Dis 1996; 22:322-328.

RETHINK TKR'S

Had total knee replaced because of pain,

Yet redness and hurting came back again.

Getting steroid injections,

But what about infections?

Aspergillus would prove to be his bane.

Note: Glucocorticoids are Aspergillus growth factors,
since they diminish the ability of neutrophils and
macrophages to combat this ubiquitous fungus. The
joint tap produced 1000 WBC's, 97% monocytes. Three
cultures grew an Aspergillus species. This genus haunts
the well-being of organ and bone marrow transplant
recipients. Others receiving long-term "steroids" will
also be at risk, especially on high doses. There has been a
second recent TKR case, not on steroids, whose purulent
knee fluid grew Mycobacterium chelonae. He had been
on a prolonged course of routine antibiotics.

Ref.: Clin Infect Dis 2007; 45:687-694

CANCER AND CALCIUM

In hypercalcemia of malignancy

Height of serum calcium drives therapy.

When severe, employ zoledronate,

With some IV saline to "hydrate".

Use denosumab if it is refractory.

Note: The cellular mediation of this problem is often the activation of osteoclasts via paracrine release of various factors by tumor cells. Mild hypercalcemia (<12 mg/dl) may respond to reduced dietary calcium, mobilization, volume repletion, and stopping thiazides, $CaCO_3$, vitamin D, and lithium. Moderate levels (12-14 mg/dl) require the addition of IV zoledronate. If it is ineffective, then denosumab (an antibody against RANK ligand) may be tried. In severe hypercalcemia (>14 mg/dl) after the failure of the above therapy, hemodialysis against a zero calcium dialysate will decrease the serum calcium by 1.5 mg/dl/hour, but it is temporary and requires careful monitoring. I have not found calcitonin to be very useful.

Refs.: UpToDate; Anticancer Res 2013; 33:2981-2988.

ATAZANAVIR LITHIASIS

Young woman on treatment for HIV,

A stone blocked her ureter distally.

Urology plucked it out.

Testing erased all our doubt.

Stone crystals matched the drug perfectly.

Note: Atazanavir urolithiasis has been reported 5 times (Japan, France, U.S.). Two stones have been analyzed. One was "yellowish and 100% atazanavir"; the other contained 60% drug and 40% calcium carbonate/apatite. The stones can be large enough to block the ureter, as was the case here. Risk factors are low fluid intake, alkaline urine, drug dose and prior stone history.

Ref.: NEJM 2006; 355: 2158-2159.

TOO MUCH IMMUNOSUPPRESSION

Heart transplant suppressed maximally,

Rituxan, apheresis, IVIG.

Diarrhea was like water,

More weight loss than he oughter.

Had histoplasma on intestinal biopsy.

Note: Gastrointestinal histoplasmosis is an uncommon problem, which is rarely diagnosed in life. Virtually every GI symptom can be seen. It is often misdiagnosed as IBD (e.g. Crohn's) or malignancy, leading to inappropriate treatments. These can be harmful. Usually, progressive disseminated infection is present, which will be fatal if untreated. Amphotericin and itraconazole are effective therapies. Choice and duration of treatment depend on the severity of illness and whether AIDS is present. Careful follow-up for signs of relapse is essential after the completion of therapy.

Ref.: Am J Gastroenterol 2005; 100:220-231.

RAMSAY HUNT SYNDROME

HIV, new right deafness and ear pain,

Has a droopy mouth, food leaks out again.

Hiccups, can't swallow right,

Right eyelid won't shut tight.

"Shingles" the culprit we did ascertain.

Note: Varicella-Zoster virus is the cause of chicken pox in the young and Herpes zoster in the more mature. Zoster (shingles) is 8-10 times more frequent in people over the age of 60 years as before 60. It can be devastating in compromised hosts. When this virus involves the 7th cranial nerve, there is weakness of all of the facial muscles on one side and an ipsilateral rash in the ear canal. Other cranial nerves may be affected at the same time and cause some of the symptoms exhibited here. Recovery from facial weakness is less common than in Bell's palsy (Herpes simplex). Early treatment with acyclovir is recommended for RHS.

Ref. NEJM 2000; 342: 635-645.

CORROSIVE SUBLIMATE

Abdominal pain and hematemesis,

Necrotizing gastro-esophagitis,

His kidneys acutely failed.

The mystery was unveiled.

Sky high mercury levels did excite us.

Note: Bichloride of mercury can be bought on the internet. It is extremely corrosive to the entire GI tract (an experienced endoscopist said that he had never seen anything like it) and causes kidney injury. It is a deadly poison of our past. As little as 500 mg can be fatal. Jack London, the author, died of mercury poisoning during self-treatment of venereal disease. Oliver Wendell Holmes stated in 1860 when it was used for various ailments: "I firmly believe that if the whole of Materia Medica, as now used, could be sunk to the bottom of the sea, it would be all the better for mankind and all the worse for the fishes". Mercurous chloride (calomel) was also on that formulary and is slightly less toxic. Fortunately, the heroic efforts of Vanderbilt physicians employing hemodialysis, apheresis and 2 chelators brought this man through a stormy course. The source of the poison is under investigation.

Ref.: Nephrol Dial Transplant 1997; 12: 328-330.

FALSE POSITIVE

Fever, somnolence, and scattered rhonchi,

Arms and legs showed many petechiae.

Lived in Nashville, not the "sticks".

Test suggested it was ticks.

But mosquitos West Nile virus did supply.

Note: The initial lumbar puncture showed 60 white cells, 80% polys. Serum antibody to Rocky Mountain spotted fever was barely positive. It's carried by the dog tick. He was treated for RMSF with doxycycline. Further testing revealed a strongly positive IgM for West Nile virus (WNV), followed by a 4-fold rise in convalescent serum. This clinched the diagnosis of WNV infection. This patient was the only proven case of WNV in Davidson County, TN in 2008. This virus uses birds as a reservoir and Culex mosquitos to infect humans. There is no current therapy except supportive care.

Ref.: Ann Intern Med 2008; 149:232-241.

CAN YOU HEAR ME NOW?

Diabetic clinic but missing his ears,

Wrestled a chow dog after too many beers.

The first ear lost with one bite.

The other blown out of sight.

Ginseng hunting's not the safest of careers.

Note: This mountain man lives in the Blue Ridge country. The second ear evaporated when his black powder rifle went off unexpectedly. He volunteered for the military during VietNam but was turned down because he had too much buckshot in his head. As his endocrinologist, Charles Upchurch, commented to me: "You just can't make this stuff up".

OUT OF THE LANDFILL

Newspapers and magazines I am savin',

Plus cardboard, I'm a recycling maven.

Turn in glass bottles, metal cans,

Plastic containers of all brands.

Those who trash these are sure
misbehavin'.

Note: The town of Amherst, MA, put 789 tons of trash
into a landfill in the 1st Quarter of 2008 at a cost of $78
per ton. They recycled 214 tons (21% recycling rate) for
a gain of $154 per ton. Profits per ton recycled were:
aluminum cans $1514, mixed paper $78, newspapers/
magazines $101, and cardboard $97. The only loss
was on glass ($14 per ton). Plastic containers were not
mentioned. I believe that it is essential for all of us to
become ardent recyclers.

INCIDENTALOMA

Headache, blurred vision, and palpitations,

Takes five hypertension medications.

Pressure is high as the skies;

Adrenal mass tripled in size.

Pheo's not just in our imaginations.

Note: This patient, whose BP was difficult to control despite 5 drugs, had neither compliance issues nor cocaine use. He had a norepinephrine-secreting pheochromocytoma! The incidentally discovered adrenal mass of 2005 had grown three-fold. Adrenal masses seen on CT scans done for other reasons, so-called incidentalomas, later are found to be pheos (5%), Cushing's (5%), primary (5%) and secondary (2.5%) adrenal carcinomas, or aldosteronomas (1%). One-fourth of non-syndromic (random) pheos will have mutations in susceptibility genes: von Hippel-Lindau, MEN-2, NF-1, or succinic dehydrogenase D.

Refs. NEJM 2007; 356:601-610; NEJM 2002; 346:1459-1466.

PIGEON PD PERITONITIS

A fungal peritonitis outbreak,

Twelve CAPD patients, no mistake.

Candida all over the ward.

Origin? They had to look hard.

Bird guano on the sills, for goodness sake.

Note: This British peritoneal dialysis unit observed 12 cases of Candida parapsilosis peritonitis over 30 months. The environmental cultures grew the organism from sinks, wash basins, a pill dispenser, a janitorial trolley, and a microwave oven. After it was isolated from pigeon "guano" on the window sills, bird-proof netting was installed on all windows of the ward. This plus thorough cleansing of the facility with 1% bleach eradicated the colonization and markedly reduced the fungal peritonitis rate.

Ref.: Nephrol Dial Transplant 1992; 7: 967-969.

SKIN CANCER IN ALLOGRAFT RECIPIENTS

Cancer in transplant patients is a bad actor.

Each immunosuppressive drug is an inhibitor.

Senescence of p53 impaired,

DNA damage not repaired,

Cyclosporine or tacrolimus the greatest factor.

Note: Since my office is on the same hall as the Dermatology Clinic, I am aware of how many of our renal transplants are present, having their multiple carcinomas removed. These are chiefly squamous cell and some are metastatic. All organ transplant recipients, who are taking calcineurin inhibitors (CNI's), are potentially affected. In essence, they have developed acquired xeroderma pigmentosum. CNI's cause aberrant p53 signaling and block the ability of cells to repair DNA damage from UV radiation. This is not seen with mTOR inhibitors (sirolimus). One of my former dialysis patients received a renal allograft in 1976. He had been on CNI's. From 1995 until 2014 he had over 100 skin cancers removed and died in hospice because of biopsy-proven metastatic squamous cell carcinoma to bone. Although decreased immune surveillance and oncogenic viruses (HPV) may also play a role, allograft patients need to be on CNI-sparing regimens, if possible, and to be counseled about UV radiation exposure being kept at a minimum.

Ref.: J Am Acad Dermatol 2014; 71:359-365.

WANT TO BUY A GAMBIAN GIANT RAT ?

Eight hundred small mammals from Central
Africa

Were shipped to a distributor in North
America.

Some carried a monkeypox virus

And infected seventy two of us,

Causing fever, a diffuse rash and cephalgia.

Note: The wisdom of this importer in 2003 defies all
common sense. Monkeypox virus (MPXV) is known to
be endemic in West Africa (Ebola land) and the Congo
Basin. Rodents are the reservoir. Humans and primates are
infected by direct contact with disease-bearing animals.
Person-to-person spread is less efficient. MPXV shares
clinical features with variola, vaccinia, and cowpox (e.g.
rash) and can be severe. In 2003, 72 human cases were
reported in the U.S. Most had been exposed to pet prairie
dogs sold by the same distributor. Guess where the
African rodents were kept! Two children required ICU
care, and one person needed a corneal transplant. There
were no deaths. A frantic search by the CDC and FDA
ensued. Only 77% of the possibly infected animals were
located. These were destroyed. There have been no new
cases since 2003. Importation of African rodents has been
prohibited. End of story?

Refs.: J Infect Dis 2006; 194:773-780; Emerg Infect Dis 2006;
12:1827-1833.

ACUTE PANCREATITIS

Epigastric pain radiates to the back.

It can mimic an acute heart attack.

Vomiting and nausea,

Fever and anorexia,

Ethanol, gall stones and drugs may interact.

Note: This common malady accounts for a quarter million hospital admissions in the U.S. every year. There are many associated conditions besides the above ones. ERCP is an iatrogenic cause. Serum lipase and abdominal CT scan are useful tests. Severe pancreatitis is defined by the failure of other organs. Scoring systems have been developed to predict severity. Careful monitoring is used, with IV fluids and nutritional support, and reimaging if things are not going well. Surgical intervention is indicated only in those with infected pancreatic necrosis. Early surgery (first few days) carries a high mortality. Antibiotics have also not been shown to be generally useful.

Refs.: NEJM 2006; 354:2142-2150; Proc Am Thorac Soc 2004; 1:289-290; BMJ 2004; 328:1407.

ACUTE PERICARDITIS

A rubbing sound brought about by friction,

PR depression and ST elevation,

And sharp, pleuritic chest pain

Echocardiogram helps explain.

Its scourge is tamponade or constriction.

Note: Inflammation of the pericardium can present
as an isolated finding or as part of a systemic illness.
In a study from Italy there were 28 cases per 100,000
population each year. It represented 5% of non-
ischemic chest pain sufferers. This is the most common
cardiac disease in HIV/AIDS. A cause is not found
in most patients. The clinical findings are a friction
rub associated with the cardiac cycle (it's scratchy or
squeaky), pleuritic chest pain eased by leaning forward/
sitting up, changes in the EKG, and/or a pericardial
effusion seen on imaging. About one third have serum
troponin elevations and are called myopericarditis. The
major acute complication is tamponade, and chronic
constriction may occur. Arrhythmias are uncommon and
mainly happen in those with underlying cardiac disease.

Refs: Curr Opin Cardiol 2012; 27:308-317; NEJM 2003;
349:684-690.

IT'S POSITIVELY UNAMERICAN

From Lone Star tick bites which alpha-gal secrete,

Specific IgE against all red meat.

Hamburger urticaria,

Pork chop angioedema,

Anaphylaxis if fried bacon you eat.

Note: It is the most common etiology of patients with anaphylaxis or episodic urticaria/angioedema for whom a causative food is discovered. "It is unusual that it is due to specific IgE against an oligosaccharide, not a protein as in most food allergy" (Dr. Rob Valet). There is a delay of 3-6 hours after ingestion of red meat (beef , pork, lamb, or cow's milk). Turkey, chicken, and fish do not cause reactions in affected patients. Galactose-alpha-1,3 galactose (alpha-gal) is the antigen. It is commonly expressed in non-primate mammalian proteins. This phenomenon is only prevalent in areas where the Lone Star tick is distributed. They have alpha-gal in their GI tracts, as does an Ixodes species in Europe, where similar allergies are found. Cross-reaction of this same IgE is the reason for anaphylaxis to cetuximab, often on the first dose, which has alpha-gal in its heavy chain. The above foods must be avoided by these unfortunate few with this allergy.

Refs.: J Allergy Clin Immunol 2009; 123:426-433; NEJM 2008; 358: 1109-1117.

VIRAL NEPHROPATHY IN ALLOGRAFTS

There is a "new" virus designated BK,

Which causes renal transplants to go astray.

Bleeding bladders in BMT's,

Wasn't seen before the mid-nineties.

Immune suppression must decrease right away.

Note: Most of the U.S. population has antibody to BK virus. Infection is thought to occur early in life. The nephropathy has a characteristic pathology, which could not have been missed in renal biopsies of transplanted patients. This was first seen in 1996 on both sides of the Atlantic. It occurs in the kidneys and bladders of other allografted patients as well. In renal transplants there was a 12.5% incidence and graft loss of 3% in one study. Plasma viral load is now available, but may underestimate the diagnosis of BK nephropathy. It is useful in follow-up. There is no licensed anti-polyoma virus therapy. Reduced immunosuppression is required. Tacrolimus et al are switched to moderate dose cyclosporine plus prednisone at this center.

Refs.: Transpl Infect Dis 2013 Nov 12 (Epub ahead of print); Transpl Int 2013; 26:822-32; BMC Nephrol 2013; 14:207.

GRIM REAPING

The vultures of India have been dying

Because the vets a new drug were trying.

Diclofenac for cattle

Gave the vultures death rattle

From uric acid excretion denying.

Note: Hindus are 80% of the Indian population and
consider cattle sacred. When one dies, it is left and eaten
by vultures. In the 1990's scientists there noticed a rapidly
decreasing vulture population (by 97%). The above
NSAID was being used by veterinarians to treat arthritis
and fever in cattle. In a careful series of experiments
it was proven that diclofenac was causing kidney
failure from uric acid retention in the vultures. Drastic
consequences included proliferation of wild dogs and
rats. Rabies from dog bites is now causing 30,000 human
deaths per year in India. The use of NSAIDs in cattle has
now been banned. Although recent data indicate some
recovery of the vulture population, the overall cost has
been estimated at 34 billion dollars.

Ref.: The Peregrine Fund – Asian Vulture Crisis.

HE WANTED MORE ENERGY

Given liothyronine for depression,

Dose was doubled at last treatment session.

In two weeks he was dyspneic.

Heart was skipping and tachycardic.

For atrial flutter we made intercession.

Rec.: The dose of 25 mcg was increased to 50 mcg daily.
Free T4 was low and TSH was undetectable. There was
2:1 block with a ventricular rate of 145 BPM. The patient
was overtly hyperthyroid. Diltiazem was begun in the
ED, and he converted to sinus rhythm. The liothyronine
was stopped, and he was changed to metoprolol.
Amiodarone was avoided. He left feeling much better,
with close follow-up. Psychiatry was notified. There is a
growing problem of "internet-enabled" and iatrogenic
hyperthyroidism. Among things being treated with or
without an M.D. are obesity, depression, weakness,
menstrual disorders, infertility, fatigue, and goiters.
A patient-directed web site called "Stop the Thyroid
Madness" advocates patients take a minimum of 3-5
grains of dessicated porcine thyroid daily for "obvious
hypothyroid symptoms", such as the above. Certain
herbals have T4 in them.

Refs.: Ann Intern Med 2009; 150:60-61; Arch Intern Med
2005; 165:831.

NEONATAL TYPE 1 DIABETES MELLITUS

One month old with "rule out septicemia",

Had DKA and hyperkalemia.

No antibody to insulin,

Had a KCNJ mutation

Cured by starting a sulfonylurea.

Note: This syndrome is rare but was diagnosed locally in two in vitro fertilization babies from the same sperm donor. It is caused by activating mutations in KCNJ11, which encodes the Kir6.2 subunit of the ATP-sensitive potassium channel. This causes 30-58% of cases of diabetes in patients under 6 months of age. They present as severe hyperglycemia and/or ketoacidosis and receive insulin. Impaired insulin secretion results from the beta-cell K(ATP) channel failing to close in response to increased intracellular ATP. Sulfonylureas close the K(ATP) channel by an ATP-independent route. In the cited study 44 of 49 (90%) consecutive patients were able to stop insulin after starting sulfonylureas.

Ref.: NEJM 2006; 355:467-477.

NEUROLEPTIC   TOXICITY

Patients with delirium and agitation,

Rigidity, high fever, and confusion.

Causes include chlorpromazine,

Haloperidol or fluphenazine.

Stop drugs and stabilize for abrogation.

Note: Neuroleptic malignant syndrome
(NMS) is a clinical diagnosis in a minority of
patients taking common psychiatric agents (the
above or clozapine, quetiapine, risperidone,
olanzapine, paliperidone and thioridazine).
Antiemetics may also be responsible
(domperidone, droperidol, promethazine,
prochlorperazine, and metoclopramide).
Mortality results from dysautonomia
(dysrhythmias, tachycardia, labile blood
pressure), hyperthermia, rhabdomyolysis, and
acute kidney injury. "Lead-pipe rigidity" can
be striking. We recently reversed NMS within
24 hours in a 91 year-old with dementia, who
was taking haloperidol, by cessation of the
drug and giving IV fluids. Attention to severe
hyperthermia, dysrhythmias and hypotension
may be needed in some patients. The course
may be "malignant" but cancer is not a factor.

Refs.: Am J Psychiatry 2007; 164:870-876; J Am Soc
Nephrol 1994; 4:1406-1412.

SEVERE   HYPERNATREMIA

Blind, under total care by his family,

Mumbling more, recent falls, sodium 203.

Dilute IV's done with caution,

He was not helped by hydration.

It was cerebral amyloid angiopathy.

Note: Although often without symptoms, cerebral
amyloid angiopathy (CAA) is an important cause of
primary lobar intracerebral bleeds in the elderly. The
prevalence at autopsy is 2.3% (ages 65-74), 8.0% (ages
75-84), and 12.1% (ages >84). The amyloid is similar
to that of Alzheimer's plaques, amyloid beta peptide.
CAA is responsible for 20% of spontaneous intracerebral
hemorrhages. Only half of subjects are demented. A
definitive diagnosis would require a tissue examination.
However, when there are 2 or more bleeds in the cortex
or gray-white junction, a probable diagnosis may be
made. Bleeds are usually recurrent. All anticoagulants
are to be avoided, including antiplatelet agents.
Treatment is supportive. This was the highest serum
sodium that I have seen.

 Refs.: Ann Neurol 2011; 70:871-880; UpToDate.

WEAKNESS AND FATIGUE

Two lung nodules, was one a carcinoma?

Swollen face, mediastinal mass, a lymphoma?

Infection was excluded.

SVC was occluded.

Biopsy showed a malignant thymoma.

Note: Thymomas are not common and usually present with thoracic symptoms, such as pain, dyspnea, cough, hoarseness, superior vena cava (SVC) syndrome, phrenic nerve compression, or pericardial effusion. Only 7% have metastases at the time of diagnosis. Myasthenia gravis, due to interference with acetylcholine receptors, is the most frequent paraneoplastic complication (30-40% of cases). It was not present in this man. He also had a moderate-sized pericardial effusion, which was assumed to be part of Stage 4 disease. At age 72 he was not offered thymectomy. Palliative chemotherapy was begun.

Ref.: Mayo Clin Proc 1993; 68:1110-1123; UpToDate.

BEWARE CYP3A4 INHIBITORS

H. pylori seen, placed on a macrolide.

Was taking a statin, other meds. beside.

Recovering from rhabdo,

Tachycardic, got amio.

CK erupted like a rising tide.

Note: The original rhabdomyolysis was mild (CK 6900, serum creatinine 2.0) and was due to the interaction of clarithromycin with simvastatin. Both drugs were stopped. As the patient improved (CK 1400), amiodarone was added to control SVT in the presence of aortic stenosis. The CK skyrocketed to 46,000 within 3 days. Acute kidney injury resulted, requiring 2 dialyses. This was my first experience with drug-interaction-related rhabdomyolysis recurring during one hospitalization. Amiodarone and clarithromycin are both CYP3A4 inhibitors. I believe that all 3 drugs contributed to episode #2.

Refs.: Drug Safety 2008; 31:587-596; Ann Intern Med 2014; 161:242-248.

HEARTLAND VIRUS

Rural dweller had confusion, myalgia,

High fever, low platelets, leukopenia.

Recently pulled off a tick.

Doxycycline did not click.

He died of overwhelming toxemia.

Note: In June 2009 two patients, who lived on farms in NW Missouri, developed a severe febrile illness after tick bites. The Lone Star tick was the likely vector for a new phlebovirus. All tests for rickettsiae and other pathogens were negative. The CDC later found that both men had viremia on day 2 of hospitalization, one week after illness began. They slowly recovered and 2 years later had serum antibody titers to the virus, which were greater than 6400. The local case was an 80 year old man, who died of a similar illness in 9-13. The persistence of an intern in pathology, who sent autopsy samples to the CDC, led to the correct diagnosis. "Tick-borne illness unresponsive to doxycyline" got the CDC's attention.

Ref.: NEJM 2012; 367:834-841.

HEART   VALVE   HEMOLYSIS

Heart valves can cause red cell fragmentation.

A foreign surface and shear stress combination,

With pressure gradient gain,

And schistocytes on blood stain.

A quick diagnosis leads to revitalization.

Note: The relationship between vascular lesions and red cell fragmentation was first described in 1962. My initial case concerned a Starr-Edwards (ball in a cage) prosthetic mitral valve. Typical lab values show anemia, increased indirect bilirubin and reticulocytes, decreased platelets, and obvious schistocytes. These sheared red cells can be seen in normal subjects at less than 0.5% (mean 0.05%) of the total red cells. Leaky or distorted prosthetic aortic or mitral valves are a common cause. Valve replacement or re-repair in 31 of 32 patients with malfunctioning mitral prostheses resulted in resolution of hemolysis. Presentation was usually within 3 months of the initial surgery. There were 2 deaths. Actuarial survival was 85% at 5 years.

Ref.: Ann Thorac Surg 2004; 77:191-195.

DON'T SUPPRESS YOUR COUGH

An older woman with bronchiectasis,

Was thin and had mild kyphoscoliosis.

To make a good impression

Had habitual cough suppression.

Her lungs harbored a mycobacteriosis.

Note: Mistakenly termed the Lady Windermere syndrome, this clinical entity is most common in elderly women. It affects the right middle lobe and lingula, because their anatomy leads to pooled respiratory secretions. Fastidious, oversensitive subjects do not want to cough, especially in the presence of others. The resultant chronic inflammation slowly destroys the bronchi and causes a vicious cycle of more secretions, worse pooling, and secondary infection. Obviously, the feeling of a need to cough will also heighten. Most have never smoked and do not have COPD. Mycobacterium avium complex (MAC) is often the pathogen. This patient had bronchoscopy, and BAL fluid grew MAC. She received clarithromycin, rifampin and ethambutol for two years with significant improvement and no major side effects. This problem is also called "atussis nervosa".

Ref.: Clin Infect Dis 2000; 30:572-575.

COLOVESICAL FISTULA

A complication of inflammation or cancer,

Urine infection and gut disease concur.

They may have pneumaturia

Or sometimes fecaluria.

Persistence will pay off with the right answer.

Note: This is a surprising enigma as illustrated by my report below (1989). It is not uncommon, as I diagnosed 2 cases in one month. Diverticulitis, Crohn's colitis, and colon or bladder cancer are common causes. Men are more often affected (71% in one series). Symptoms are varied and may be absent or overlooked without direct questioning. Pneumaturia, abdominal pain, and dysuria are seen in 55-67%. A typical patient presents with fever, an abdominal mass, and recurrent cystitis, but no bowel-related symptoms. A cystogram is the best test, but can be negative. So keep looking if you suspect this problem. Surgical correction can be challenging and may require at least a two-stage procedure.

Refs.: J Urol 1978; 119:744-746; J Urol 1989; 142:815-816.

LIGHT CHAIN-LIMITED MYELOMA

No symptoms despite his uremia,

The lab tests showed hypercalcemia.

Whole immunoglobulins low,

Serum lambda light chains did show.

A lung mass was a plasmacytoma.

Note: A study of 1027 myeloma patients at the Mayo Clinic found that 16% had only a lambda or a kappa light chain (LC) as the paraprotein. Such cases often present with renal disease, in my experience. The serum immunofixation will show a LC band if the GFR is decreased enough. The serum free LC ratio will also be altered. Most often the renal biopsy demonstrates cast nephropathy. Recently, the Mayo group has been able to define a LC MGUS by using the serum free LC ratio. It was found in 0.8% of 18 thousand local residents over 50 years old. This represented 19% of total MGUS patients. Risk of progression to myeloma was 0.3 per 100 patient-years (better prognosis) vs. 1.0 in conventional MGUS. Of 129 patients with LC MGUS, 23% had renal disease.

Refs.: Mayo Clin Proc 2003; 78:21-33; Lancet 2010; 375:1721-1728; Am J Clin Pathol 2009; 131:166-171.

LEMIERRE SYNDROME

Healthy young man with recent pharyngitis,

Now has jugular thrombophlebitis,

Lungs and joints with abscesses.

Blood gram negatives expresses.

Mouth anaerobes sneaking in to bite us.

Note: A middle-aged man with 3-4 weeks of fever, weight loss and right-sided weakness had brain and liver abscesses on imaging. He had self-treated "the flu" several weeks earlier. Risk factors for complications were smoking, decayed teeth, alcoholism and a colovesical fistula. Fusobacterium nucleatum grew from his liver abscess, but not his blood (prior antibiotics). Lemierre syndrome is typically characterized by oropharyngeal infection, metastatic abscesses, Fusobacterium septicemia and frequently by involvement of the internal jugular vein. F. necrophorum is the usual pathogen, but F. nucleatum is second. Treatment starts with 6 weeks of antibiotics and may require abscess drainage. Survival is amazingly good since many subjects were in prior good health, unlike the cited case, whose teeth had to be pulled. The poem is about a classic case in a previously healthy young man.

Refs.: Rev Infect Dis 1989; 11:319-324; Medicine 1989; 68:85-94.

LABORATORY-ACQUIRED INFECTIONS

Bacteria cause these most commonly.

Dimorphic fungi contribute, plus HIV.

There are thousands to protect;

Their welfare we mustn't neglect.

Better safety has reduced cases importantly.

Note: There are an estimated 500,000 lab workers in the U.S. They are exposed to a variety of organisms, especially those who work in microbiology. In a review of 4,079 cases, 159 agents were implicated, but 10 accounted for >50% of infections. Bacteria made up 43%, with Brucellae the most frequent (RR=8,013) and Neisseria meningitidis next (RR=41). Shigellae, Salmonellae, and TB are also common. Cultures from tularemia patients are dangerous. Inhalational exposure to conidia of histoplasmosis, blastomycosis and coccidioidomycosis account for most of the fungal infections. Hepatitis B and C, alongwith HIV, are the major viral agents. Parasites are rare. Physicians must take a careful occupational history in febrile patients. There also needs to be an improved system of reporting these cases. RR=relative risk versus a normal population.

Refs.: Health Lab Sci 1976; 13:105-114; Clin Infect Dis 2009; 49:142-147.

SEVERE HYPONATREMIA

Slowly down to one hundred it decreased.

Psych medicine and HCTZ had not ceased.

BUN and creat. were low;

Urine osm. wasn't apropos.

Sodium level must be carefully increased.

Note: This patient's lab tests best fit a diagnosis of SIADH. He was taking a haloperidol cousin for bipolar disorder and PTSD. It has caused SIADH. Hydrochlorthiazide (HCTZ) blocks urinary dilution by inhibiting the NaCl cotransporter in the distal convoluted tubule of the nephron in a dose-related manner. Patients with a high liquid intake are susceptible to hyponatremia from either mechanism. Markers of SIADH in routine blood work are low concentrations of BUN, creatinine and urate due to mild volume expansion from enhanced water retention. Therapy with IV isotonic saline will fail because urine osmolality is fixed in the 400-600 range. The best treatment is cessation of offending drugs and liquid restriction to <1 liter/day. In emergencies, hypertonic saline or ADH inhibitors may be used. Serum Na should not rise more than 0.5 meq/l/hour.

Refs.: Clin J Am Soc Nephrol 2008; 3:1175-84; Ann Intern Med 1989; 110:24-30.

INTESTINAL ANGINA

A heavy smoker with bad abdominal pain,

Weight loss because from food he did abstain.

Both a negative EGD

And a colonoscopy.

An arteriogram the symptoms did explain.

Note: Diffuse atherosclerosis affected all three major bowel arteries. The SMA and IMA were nearly totally occluded. The proximal celiac artery was 60% closed. He had lost 30 lbs. of obese weight over 3 months due to post-prandial periumbilical and epigastric pain. This pain is usually dull and crampy, occurring in the first hour after eating. A bland diet does not help. Fatty foods and big meals make it worse. Other atherosclerotic syndromes are often present. In the operating room prosthetic grafts have lower morbidity and mortality than vein grafts. Poor surgical candidates may be treated with percutaneous transluminal angioplasty or stents.

Refs.: Ann Vasc Surg 2012; 26:447-453; Arch Intern Med 2006; 166:2095-2100.

EMBOLIC ENDOCARDITIS

Twenty two year-old with severe head pain,

High polys in CSF we needed to explain.

In rehab for pain pill abuse,

Brain imaging with changes diffuse,

The echocardiogram came through again.

Note: This young man was a parenteral and intranasal
oxycodone user. A systolic murmur was heard.
Neurologic exam was normal. His temperature was
102 degrees. A peripheral blood WBC was 16.4 K with
89% neutrophils. The CSF WBC was 960 with 86%
neutrophils. Blood culture was slowly growing gram
positive cocci. The mitral valve had a 3x2x4 cm mass
on echo. Valve surgery was planned. A consecutive
series of 214 patients with infective endocarditis, who
required cardiac surgery, was followed for up to 20 years
in Austria. In 65 patients verified stroke occurred. Fifty
of 65 survived surgery (82%). They had poorer survival
than non-stroke patients. Complete neurologic recovery
was seen in 35 (70% of survivors), but MCA stroke did
less well. This patient's MRI showed several strokes.

Ref.: Stroke 2006; 37:2094-2099.

ACETAMINOPHEN
(APAP, PARACETAMOL)

The most poorly regulated drug toxin,

It's contained in a host of medication.

The FDA this would avert;

Pharmacists are on the alert.

Doctors must ramp up patient education.

Note: This popular drug is produced by the ton and is part of greater than 600 prescription and over-the-counter (OTC) products in the U.S. Up to 78,000 ED visits and 34,000 hospitalizations occur each year from APAP toxicity. There are uncounted deaths, chiefly from acute liver failure, which is dose-related. Half of these are unintentional. At UT Southwestern it is estimated that a single dose of 12-16 grams is enough to kill 50% of adults. Unbelievably to me, a daily adult dose of 4 grams is thought to be safe. Children and alcoholics are more susceptible. Physicians need to ask users of OTC APAP: what size bottle, what tablet strength, how long does a bottle last and do they have prescribed APAP?

Refs.: ACP Internist May 2014, p.14; Medicine 1997; 76:185-191.

RELAPSING FEVER IN MURFREESBORO

A woman with cough, fever, and myalgia,

She was treating new calves with diarrhea.

Family members were affected.

The cultures nothing detected.

This microbe was first found in Australia.

Note: Coxiella burnetii is the cause of a zoonosis that is world-wide. It's a "sturdy organism" with high infectivity and prolonged survival in the environment. It shouldn't be grouped with rickettsiae and varies widely in cases per million population per year (France 500; Australia 38; U.S. 0.28). Pets and ruminants are the biggest sources. A cat giving birth under a poker table infected 12 people in the same room. Acute illnesses are mainly mild pneumonia and hepatitis. Chronic infections often cause "culture-negative" endocarditis. The pathogen does not grow on standard media. Diagnosis requires antibody titers or PCR/immunohistology of tissue. Treatment of acute illness is 2 weeks of doxycycline. Endocarditis is treated with long courses of doxycycline and hydroxychloroquine.

Ref.: Mayo Clin Proc 2008; 83:574-579.

41

RIGHT SHOULDER PAIN

Awoke five days before with shoulder
hurting,

Malaise, dizziness, fever, and not eating.

Lab work showed rapid hemolysis,

AKI and leukocytosis.

On his back a brown recluse had been
biting.

Note: Necrotic lesions caused by the bite of Loxosceles
reclusa are common in the South. This spider is
large, tan and has the image of a fiddle on its back.
Sphingomyelinase D in the venom causes structural
damage to the skin and can have systemic effects.
Hemolysis is complement-mediated and can be delayed
for 5-7 days. It was fatal to a 3 year-old girl at Vanderbilt
in 2010. Treatment is supportive, with RBC transfusions
as needed. This 60 year-old required 7 units of RBCs
to keep his HCT in the low 20's. The skin lesion has
a necrotic center and should be kept clean, but not
debrided or biopsied. Recovery of the skin is slow.

Refs.: Am J Clin Pathol 1995; 104:463-467; J Am Acad
Dermatol 2001; 44:561-573; Ann Emerg Med 2012;
60:439-441.

THIAZIDES AND ETHANOL

Alcoholic with mouth sores, who could not eat,

Beer and water intake he cannot excrete.

Serum sodium 108,

Mental status not doing great,

Slow saline correction got him on his feet.

Note: Ingestion of dilute fluids without solute (Na, K, Cl, and urea from metabolism) leads to hyponatremia, which can be extreme and even fatal. At least 50 mosms of solute per liter of water ingested are required for urinary secretion. Beer has none. Furthermore, thiazide diuretics (HCTZ, metolazone, chlorthalidone, et al) prevent the kidneys from diluting the urine. A dozen 12 ounce cans a beer per day (not an unusual intake) contain 4.3 liters of water. Thus, 215 mosms of solute would be needed to excrete this volume (e.g. 215 meq of NaCl). Counsel alcoholics about rehab and about the choice of a diuretic/antihypertensive which isn't a thiazide. They should eat a balanced diet containing protein and not excessive NaCl. Food fadists are also susceptible to this syndrome, in that they shun salt and animal protein.

Refs.: J Am Soc Nephrol 2008; 19:1076-1078; Clin Nephrol 1996; 45:61-64; Am J Kidney Dis 1998; 31:1028-1031.

COXSACKIE MYOPERICARDITIS

A young woman with fever and pleuritic
pain,

Her heart was pounding like an express
train.

A large left pleural effusion,

Cardiac shadow was swollen,

It was infection from an enterovirus strain.

Note: This 26 year-old school teacher was previously
healthy, but had a 2 year-old and was newly pregnant.
She had been ill for 2 weeks with chest pain and dyspnea
(even at rest). A large pleural and moderate pericardial
effusions were found. Testing was positive for Coxsackie
B4. Enteroviruses are transmitted by the fecal-oral
route and typically may affect both the myocardium
and pericardium. The group B coxsackieviruses are
the most frequent cause of myocarditis in the U.S. and
Western Europe. Most enteroviral infections during
pregnancy are mild and do not result in fetal disease or
miscarriage. Good hygiene by the mother is protective,
especially for those with other youngsters. This patient
had a pericardiocentesis and recovered uneventfully.

Refs.: Br Heart J 1966; 28:204-220; UpToDate.

ESOPHAGEAL ADENOCARCINOMA

Sixty three year-old with odynophagia,

Weight loss from poor intake and dysphagia.

CT of the distal esophagus

Showed nodes and increased thickness.

Prognosis is poor for this neoplasia.

Note: Esophageal cancer is a very aggressive malignancy. Adenocarcinoma is increasing in frequency in the U.S. Barrett's esophagus is a risk factor, but only 1% progress to adenocarcinoma each year. Other risk factors are obesity, white race, smoking, alcoholism, and reflux. Dysphagia and unintentional weight loss are typical symptoms. Metastases, as here, are often found at presentation. Despite advances in surgical technique and chemotherapy, there is only a 14% five-year survival. Targeted therapeutic agents are in development, but few are approved so far. HER-2 inhibitors lead the list for metastatic disease. VEGF, COX-2, mTOR, and EGFR are pathways under investigation.

Refs.: NEJM 2011; 365:1375-1383; World J Gastroenterol 2015; 21:7933-7943; Can Assoc Radiol 2015; 66:130-139.

RESPIRATORY SYNCYTIAL VIRUS (RSV)

A virus with a seasonal incidence

Kids catch it by their third year of existence.

URI, bronchiolitis,

Otitis, or pneumonitis,

Immunosuppressed need special vigilance.

Note: RSV and the parainfluenza viruses are the chief cause of hospitalization for respiratory illness in young children. These occur in a 22 week period from November to April. Dispersed by aerosolized secretions from infected children or adults, the incubation is 2-8 days in the nasopharynx, with spread to the lungs 1-3 days later. Severe illness is less common in adults unless they are compromised hosts. Wheezing, rhonchi, decreased leukocytosis, and less fever separate RSV from bacterial pneumonia in adults, while infiltrates on chest films look the same. Isolation and banning visitors with URIs are useful strategies. Ribavirin is effective if started early. Oral ribavirin is as good as having it inhaled in adults and less costly. Vaccines have not worked thus far.

Refs.: NEJM 2001; 344:1917-28; NEJM 2009; 360:588-98; J Heart Lung Transplant 2012; 31:839-44.

PAGET DISEASE OF BONE

Nine per cent of the elderly are afflicted,

With bone pain and deformity inflicted.

Get plain films when seniors present;

Nuclear scans show the extent.

Patient function may become restricted.

Note: PDB develops in the elderly (>55 years) from genetic (seven genes identified) and environmental influences. Although many are asymptomatic, excessive bone remodeling results in abnormal deposition of lamellar bone interspersed with woven bone. Bone volume is increased, and marrow is replaced with stromal tissue. Symptoms include pain, arthritis, deformity, pathologic fracture, and loss of functional status. Involved areas are skull, thoracolumbar spine, pelvis and long bones of the legs. Diagnosis is primarily radiologic. Serum alkaline phosphatase (SAP) is usually elevated. My patient, who fractured his left femoral neck by just getting into his car, had an SAP which was almost five times the ULN. He had no liver disease to account for the high SAP, but the diagnosis of PDB was only made then. Hypercalcemia, hypercalciuria and renal stones may be seen occasionally. Treatment with nitrogen-containing bisphosphonates is recommended (Grade 1A). Zoledronic acid is infused IV every 6 months.

Refs.: NEJM 2005; 353:898-908; UpToDate.

SCABIES

A skin rash caused by an arachnid mite,

Diffuse, intense itching that is worse at night.

It's spread by skin-to-skin contact;

Shared clothes may also interact.

Immunosuppressed have a dreadful plight.

Note: Sarcoptes scabiei completes its entire life cycle in humans. Only females burrow into the skin. Males wander around. The mites are invisible to the naked eye. A skin eruption begins in 3-6 weeks as a combination of infestation and hypersensitivity. However, hosts are able to transmit the infection while asymptomatic. Lesions develop in finger webs, flexor surfaces of the wrists, elbows, axillae, buttocks, genitalia, and female breasts. Severe pruritus ensues (it's worse at night). Immunosuppressed subjects (e.g. HIV) have much larger populations of mites (many thousands) , causing thick, crusted areas. Any infestation requires aggressive treatment of not only all contacts and household members, but also the environment. Topical permethrin and lindane are effective for individuals. Ivermectin is a safe and effective oral agent.

Ref.: NEJM 2006; 354:1718-1727; Am J Med 2009; 122:632-635 (eosinophilia mentioned).

EBOLA   VIRUS

Hemorrhagic fever now in West Africa,

Outbreaks started from a sick primate area.

Then it was spread person-to-person,

Quickly became a health care burden

In Sierra Leone, Guinea and Liberia.

Note: Ebola is one of 2 filovirus genera. Marburg is
the other. They are highly transmissible by direct
contact with or body fluids from an infected human or
ape. Using sick primates as a food source is one way.
Within 1-2 weeks a severe illness begins with fever,
chills, weakness, headache, muscle pain, cough and
GI symptoms. Worsening prostration, stupor, and
hypotension ensue. Signs of impaired coagulation,
liver dysfunction from necrosis, and cytopenias are
seen. Isolation and protection of medical personnel
are imperative. Treatment is supportive, and there
is no vaccine. At last count there have been 888 cases
in the current outbreak with a 61% mortality. Small
animals, especially bats, are thought to be the reservoir.
Vanderbilt was awarded a large federal grant in 2013 to
study treatment and prevention (Dr. James Crowe, PI).

Ref.: Lancet 2011; 377;849-862; NEJM 2014; 371:2092-
2100.

THE FORMER ENTEROBACTER SAKAZAKII

Cronobacter can cause newborn colitis

And severe neonatal meningitis.

It is a gram-negative rod,

Found in most food, home and abroad.

Our man had bacteremic cholangitis.

Note: This organism is a significant risk to the health of neonates. It is an emerging opportunistic pathogen which causes necrotizing enterocolitis, meningitis, and sepsis in premature and full-term infants. Those aged less than 28 days are at greatest risk. Powdered infant formula (unsterile) has been implicated. Good hygiene is needed in its preparation. Breast feeding avoids this issue. However, this organism has been isolated from a wide variety of foods cited in a reference below. Adult cases are rare. As of 2007 there were only 10 cases in the literature. Most were immunocompromised. Our patient was a previously healthy 89 year old with cholangitis and a negative ERCP. He responded well to antibiotics.

Refs.: Clin Infect Dis 2006; 42:996-1002; Age Ageing 2007; 36:595-6; Int J Food Microbiol 2007; 116:1-10.

IT SOUNDS LIKE AN ASIAN ENTRÉE

There is a new virus called chikungunya.

Aedes mosquitos live here, might have
stung ya.

Headache, myalgias, arthritis,

Pink rash and conjunctivitis,

Be sure they're well before they come out
among ya.

Note: This is an acute, debilitating arboviral disease
of Asia and Africa. Aedes mosquitos transmit it
and are found in all TN counties. Infected travelers
from endemic areas are the main source of resident
Tennesseans becoming infected. The traveler transmits
it to local mosquitos. Timely diagnosis, isolation
of infected individuals, and alerting public health
departments are critical in quelling outbreaks. In the
summer of 2007, 337 cases occurred in the area of
Bologna/Ravenna, Italy. Thus far in 2014 there have
been 12 cases in TN. Diagnosis is based on signs and
symptoms. Testing serum or CSF for virus-specific IgM
confirms it. Treatment is supportive. The name of this
virus means "bent over in pain".

Refs.: Ann Glob Health 2014; 80:466-475; www.cdc.gov/
chikungunya.

COBALT CARDIOMYOPATHY

A middle-aged woman whose health went to pieces,

Dyspnea of heart failure steadily increases.

LVAD and transplant entailing,

Then the allograft was failing.

A disaster caused by her joint prostheses.

Note: In 1966 a new syndrome of fulminant heart failure appeared in Quebec City, Canada. The victims were heavy beer drinkers, who used a brand to which cobalt chloride had been added to preserve the foam. Pericardial effusions were part of the illness. A confirmatory study in Minneapolis soon followed. The subjects had an average age in the 40's and drank beer with cobalt in it. The mortality was 43%. Both reports emphasized that this illness differed from ethanol or beriberi heart disease. It also could be reversed with cobalt removal. Cobalt use in food was banned here in 1966. An exceptional recent case of cardiomyopathy causing fulminant heart failure requiring desperate measures appeared in the NEJM, and was only figured out when the prosthetic joints were recalled. The serum cobalt level was 288 mcg/liter (normal <1.0). When the hip prostheses were both removed, the patient started to recover well being.

Refs.: Am J Med 1972; 53:395-417; NEJM 2014; 370:559-566.

MARFAN SYNDROME

Long arms and legs, aortic root dilation,

Half of them under 40 years with dissection,

Joint hypermobility,

Lenses displaced upwardly,

Angiotensin blockade leads to life extension.

Note: Marfan syndrome (MFS) is an autosomal dominant disorder causing premature death. Most subjects have mutations in the fibrillin-1 gene and an affected parent. One quarter have new mutations. A mutant TGF-beta receptor afflicts a minority. The MFS phenotype is quite variable and can affect multiple organs. The aorta is dilated (but less elastic) in 50% of children with MFS. This is progressive. Complications include aortic valve regurgitation and aortic dissection with rupture (the cause of death in 80%). Other features include ectopia lentis, long arms and legs (compared to torso length), arachnodactyly, joint laxity (thumb sign), and scoliosis. In a study of 18 pediatric patients with MFS by Dietz et al, ARB therapy reduced the rate of aortic root dilation by 7-fold. Noncanonical signaling by TGF-beta is felt to be the cause of aortic dilation.

Ref.: NEJM 2008; 358:2787-2795.

"CRYPTOGENIC"   CIRRHOSIS

Man recently found to have mutation in A1A,

Misfolded protein in liver cells, can't get away.

Panacinar emphysema,

ZZ allele is anathema.

This also predisposes to GPA.

Note: The combination of hepatic cirrhosis and emphysema conjures up either smokers with alcoholism or with HCV. However, one should not forget hereditary alpha1-antitrypsin (A1A) deficiency . Although one allele comes from each parent, the more Z you have, the worse the disease (95% of afflicted subjects are ZZ). If this protein malfunctions, the proteinases generated by lung inflammation aren't degraded, gradually destroying the distal acini. Smoking plus ZZ causes emphysema to appear 19 years earlier. In the liver, the misfolded protein cannot exit and causes hepatocyte death, resulting in fibrosis. Granulomatous polyangiitis (GPA) has also been linked to A1A deficits, because proteinase-3 is not being normally inhibited at sites of inflammation by A1A. Hepatic transplantation cures the liver aspect, but not the residual lung disease.

Refs.: NEJM 2002; 346: 45-53; NEJM 2000; 343:1933; Arthritis Rheum 2010; 62:3760-3767.

THINK OUTSIDE THE BOX

Heart transplant with renal insufficiency,

Work-up finds monoclonal gammopathy.

HOCM pre-graft diagnosis,

Different cause we must not miss,

We'll see if amyloid caused this
hypertrophy.

Note: A simple procedure, which is often not considered, is to restain pathologic tissue for a diagnosis not picked up on routine processing. A patient of mine with nephrotic syndrome and a high prothrombin time due to factor X deficiency was diagnosed with AL amyloidosis by obtaining tissue sections from a cholecystectomy at another hospital for Congo red staining. Cardiac involvement by this amyloidosis causes diastolic dysfunction, conduction problems, hypertrophy and symptomatic heart failure. The patient with "HOCM" had 410 mg/dl of an MGUS in his serum post-transplant, which was a lambda light chain. Lambda light chain is favored over kappa monoclonals in AL amyloid by a 3:1 ratio.We now await the reprocessing of the patient's original heart sections for Congo red staining.

Refs.: Arch Intern Med 2006; 166:1805-1813; Circulation 2009; 120:1203-1212.

APPENDICITIS

Abdominal pain, nausea, emesis,

At first there's inflammation, necrosis.

A good doctor does not wait,

Or else they will perforate.

CT scan's the best bet for diagnosis.

Note: There are a lot of pitfalls in some patients, which lead to a delay in diagnosis. Many other abdominal conditions can mimic it. The position of the appendiceal tip may be in 5 different areas from retrocecal to pelvic and determines the symptoms and signs. This condition occurs in 8.6% of males and 6.7% of females in a lifetime. The peak decade is 10-19 years. Perforation is to be avoided. It occurs in 10% within the first 24 hours. Of all perforations, 65% happen after 48 hours. Treatment is either open laparotomy or by an endoscopic approach. Medical therapy alone results in increased perforations and is not an option. Mortality is 0.08% in those receiving surgery.

Refs.: Ann Intern Med 2011; 154:789-796; Lancet 2011; 377:1573-79; Ann Surg 1997; 225:252-261,.

DRUG-INDUCED LUPUS (DIL)

It is not quite as difficult as the real thing.

Arthralgias, myalgias, and fatigue are troubling.

Procainamide, hydralazine,

Anti-TNFs, minocycline,

Early drug cessation leads to disease receding.

Note: This condition has been known for over 50 years and requires long-term use of about 20 common drugs. Young women taking chronic minocycline for acne is the latest cause to come to my attention. Although the pathogenesis is incompletely understood, autoimmunity is involved, as in systemic lupus. A predisposing factor in DIL is N-acetylation speed. Slow acetylation of drugs was present in 97% of patients in one study of DIL. Hydralazine has the highest incidence (5%), occurring particularly in those on larger doses for prolonged periods. When the offending drug is stopped, symptoms generally abate over days to weeks. NSAIDs will help control symptoms until then. Glucocorticoids and other immunosuppressives can be used in patients with more severe symptoms.

Refs: Arch Intern Med 1987; 147:599-600; J Rheumatol 2005; 32:740-743; NEJM 1988; 318:1431-1436; Clin Nephrol 1984; 22:230-238.

COGNITIVE DISORDERS AFTER CABG

Up to eighty per cent when tested formally,

Affects attention, motor speed, and memory.

It overlaps with delirium;

Causes include embolism.

In most patients this state resolves
gradually.

Note: Many patients undergoing coronary artery
bypass grafting (CABG) develop neurocognitive
complications, which can be subtle and first recognized
by family members. Executive function may be slow to
return. I have had several patients tell me that it took
over a month for them to be fully able to perform their
work at a preoperative level. Cerebral ischemia from
hypoperfusion during the procedure is one of the causes.
Atheroembolism, thromboembolism, and even air
embolism have occurred. Risk factors are advanced age,
the extent of proximal atherosclerosis (e.g. carotids),
prior stroke, and hypertension. Although there are long-
term complications of cognitive changes associated with
CABG, only the short-term appear to be directly related
to the operation.

Refs.: Ann Neurol 2005; 57:615-621; Semin Neurol 2006;
26:432-439.

HISTOPLASMOSIS AFTER SOLID ORGAN TRANSPLANT

Woman with renal transplant and pyrexia,

Graft was ten months old, and she had dyspnea.

No travel outside Tennessee,

Her kidney functioned normally.

The whole blood PCR revealed Histoplasma.

Note: Histoplasmosis is a disease of people who live in the river valleys of the central U.S. The organism is inhaled, can cause a flu-like illness, and then may persist without symptoms in the host. An 8-year study from 24 institutions of 152 solid organ recipients with histoplasmosis, found a median time from transplant to diagnosis of 27 months, but 34% were discovered in the first year after grafting. Organs received were: kidney (51%), liver (16%), kidney/pancreas (14%), heart (9%), lung (5%), and other (4%). Disseminated disease was seen in 81%, and 28% needed ICU care at admission. Urine Histoplasma antigen was positive in 93%. Most (73%) received initial amphotericin, with an azole continued for 12 months. Mortality was 10% and 6% relapsed.

Refs.: Clin Infect Dis 2013; 57:1542-1549; Ann Clin Lab Sci 2009; 39:409-412 (VU PCR reference).

DRUG INTERACTION HYPOGLYCEMIA

Sixteen common antibiotics were studied

In Texas Medicare patients also prescribed

An oral hypoglycemic.

Low glucose was the metric.

Five problematic agents were identified.

Note: A diabetic cohort was retrospectively studied from 2006-2009. They had filled a prescription for a common oral antibiotic used in the elderly. Rates of hypoglycemic events in the next 14 days were compared. for the 16 drugs. Five antibiotics had higher odds ratios for hypoglycemia: clarithromycin (3.96), levofloxacin (2.60), trimethoprim-sulfamethoxazole (2.56), metronidazole (2.11), and ciprofloxacin (1.62). Nine of the other 11 antimicrobials were used as the reference standard. In 2009, 28.3% of the subjects receiving either glipizide or glyburide were prescribed 1 of the 5 with higher odds ratios. This was associated with 13% of the hypoglycemic events. Hospitalization was required in 40% of these hypoglycemias, and 9 patients died. Only 3 patients died in the control group.

Refs.: JAMA Internal Medicine (online) 9-1-14; ACP Internist 2014; 34:14.

RECURRENT CLOSTRIDIUM DIFFICILE COLITIS

This infection is increasing markedly,

Antibiotic-resistant spores the enemy.

Fecal biome transplants seem vile.

Probiotics need further trial.

Doctors must figure out better therapy.

Note: During frequent ward attending months, I observe a lot of this. Failures of antibiotic-alone regimens and frequent hospitalizations are common. I have seen 2 patients rapidly develop toxic megacolon in this setting. One was set off by a PCP giving him levofloxacin for a mild respiratory illness. Spores of the organism are unaffected by antimicrobials. A sensible approach is to decrease the load of viable pathogens (and spores) using antimicrobials, and then to introduce new gut flora. Donor stool transplantation is not widely accepted. However, probiotics are being sold in many supermarkets and health food stores. Kefir is one of these. The internet can show you how to make it at home.

Refs.: Clin Infect Dis 2014; 59:858-861; Ann Intern Med 2012; 157:878-888; Ann Intern Med 2011; 155:839-847.

MIDDLE EAST RESPIRATORY SYNDROME (MERS)

This severe illness struck Saudi Arabia,

With fever, rigors, cough, and worse dyspnea.

Scary, often deadly contagion,

Risks are age, comorbid condition.

A new coronavirus inhabits this area.

Note: MERS is caused by a coronavirus named MERS-CoV. All of the cases have been linked to countries in or near the Arabian Peninsula. The outbreak began in 2012. Two patients with MERS arrived in the U.S. from Saudi Arabia in May 2014. Seventy consecutive MERS patients from Riyadh, S.A. were reviewed in October 2014. Median age - 62 years, 66% were male, and 56% were nosocomial. Fever, dyspnea, cough, and pneumonia on chest films (90%) were common findings. ICU therapy was required in 70 %. Infections came in clusters. Mortality was 60% and was higher in those over 65 years of age. Comorbidities included chronic heart disease, diabetes, hypertension and chronic renal disease. Only 4% were previously healthy. Treatment was supportive.

Refs.: Int J Infect Dis 2014, Oct 7, Saad et al (epub); Lancet Infect Dis 2013; 13:752-761; Clin Infect Dis 2014, Oct 16, Drosten et al (epub).

STREPTOCOCCUS PNEUMONIAE

Common, gram-positive diplococcus,

Pasteur and Sternberg discovered it in pus.

A breakthrough with penicillin,

The vaccine came from Austrian.

This germ is still threatening all of us.

Note: Invasive pneumococcal infections cause significant morbidity and mortality despite effective antibiotics. Pneumonitis, meningitis, bacteremia, endocarditis and otitis media lead the list. Drug-resistance is emerging. The elderly and young children are most at risk. Asplenia, chronic lung or cardiovascular disease, HIV, hematologic malignancy, and immunosuppressed states are also risk factors. A particular hero of mine is Robert Austrian, who devoted his academic life at the University of Pennsylvania to defeating this organism. One should not forget Oswald Avery, who was the first to discover DNA using the pneumococcus. Somehow the Nobel Prize committee whiffed on that one.

Refs.: J Exp Med 1944; 79:137-158; Medicine 1997; 76:295-303; Am J Med 1999; 107(1A): 12S-27S; A symposium in honor of Dr. Robert Austrian's work: Am J Med 1999; 107(1A): 1S-90S.

COMPLICATION OF MEDIASTINAL GRANULOMAS

Came in with dyspnea, cough, and hemoptysis;

CT revealed mediastinal fibrosis.

Granulomatous infection

Led to bronchial occlusion.

Tennessee has endemic histoplasmosis.

Note: Mediastinal granuloma is much more common and more benign than mediastinal fibrosis. Even though the granulomas can be large and acting as a mass, they may cause little damage and few or no symptoms. When there are symptoms, the mass is compressing compliant structures such as the superior vena cava and esophagus. However, it is a different story with mediastinal fibrosis, a less common but more serious sequela of mediastinal adenitis. A thick dense fibrotic capsule invades (not compresses) airways and even arteries. Complete obliteration can be seen. The interval between infection with an organism like Histoplasma capsulatum and fibrosis can take years. Most subjects are young adults. Therapy is difficult.

Refs.: Medicine 1988; 67:295-310; Medicine 2006; 85:37-42.

PONTIAC FEVER

They went out to eat down Opryland way

And were keen to try the trendy new café.

The mist was contaminated,

With Legionellae saturated.

Two thirds of diners caught more than the buffet.

Note: A case control study of this outbreak showed that 68% of patrons interviewed became ill with fever (100%), myalgias (93%), headache (87%), and fatigue (79%). The mean incubation period was 49 hours, with illness lasting a mean of 71 hours. A large fountain area seated 58% of afflicted persons. Legionella anisa was cultured from the fountain pool. High antibody titers to it were found in half of tested ill subjects. "Pontiac fever" was first described in1968 in Pontiac, MI. It was a lesser illness compared to pneumonic legionellosis. Flu symptoms and fever of short duration are caused by a variety of Legionella species. Inhalation of contaminated water in a number of settings has been implicated; e.g. hot tubs, spas, home hot water, outdoor showers, and potting soil. Cleaning the water system in this restaurant corrected the problem.

Refs.: Clin Infect Dis 2003; 37:1292-1297; Medicine 1989; 68:116-132.

DELIRIUM

A disturbance in awareness and attention,

An additional defect in cognition,

Which develops in hours to days.

The patient's brain is ablaze

Related to a serious medical condition.

Note: The exact pathophysiology of delirium is unknown, but it is believed to be the product of oxidative stress on the brain. This attacks the most vulnerable neurons, both dopaminergic and cholinergic. There is a hyperdopaminergic state and hypocholinergic state created. The excess dopamine potentiates the action of glutamate, an excitatory neurotransmitter. Hallucinations and agitation ensue. The lack of acetylcholine causes deficits in alertness and attention. Delirium is believed to be a permanent neurodestructive process, resulting in irreversible loss of critical neurons. Definitive therapy is to halt the initiating process. Haloperidol may be neuroprotective.

Refs.: Med Clin North Am 2010; 94:1103-1116; Ann Intern Med 2011; 154:746-751.

ACUTE PYELONEPHRITIS AND AKI

AKI is unusual in pyelonephritis.

It's not straightforward like acute cystitis.

Must rule out urinary obstruction

And realize that this situation

Needs six weeks of treatment like endocarditis.

Note: I have seen about 1-2 male patients per year with acute kidney injury (AKI) from pyelonephritis. There was not a complex scenario such as obstruction or acute tubular necrosis from sepsis due to urinary pathogens. Many were alcoholic. None were hypotensive or receiving nephrotoxic drugs. Misdiagnosis was common. Some needed a short course of hemodialysis. Recovery of renal function was often slow and marked by continued pyuria on appropriate antibiotics. Even six weeks may not be enough. One of my patients died. Autopsy showed kidneys weighing 420 and 440 grams (normal – 150 grams each), which exuded purulent material when cut. There was no anatomic obstruction. Our latest case grew out Pasteurella multocida from his blood (many cat scratches and bites).

Refs.: Am J Nephrol 1991; 11:257-259; Am J Med Sci 2004; 328:121-123; Am J Kidney Dis 1986; 8:271-273.

PERICARDIAL EFFUSIONS

There often appears to be confusion

In cases of large pericardial effusion.

One big risk is tamponade.

Experts' advice can be flawed.

Echo-guided tap is safe. It's my conclusion.

Note: With the advent of 2-D echocardiography,
the ease of diagnosis and treatment of pericardial
effusion (PE) has advanced. Chest CT scans also pick
up occasional cases. The controversy occurs when
physicians pronounce that moderate-to-large PEs don't
need to be drained. A comprehensive review of the
Mayo Clinic's experience from 1979-2000, broken into
tertiles, is instructive. Most effusions (80-83%) were
circumferential. Half were bloody, and malignancy
was the greatest cause (25-41%). In the latest group
74% of patients had tamponade, and most of these
PEs were not large (<400 ml on initial aspiration). In
75% prolonged catheter drainage was employed. This
resulted in a decrease both in recurrence rates and in
the need for surgery. There was only one death in 977
patients.

Refs.: Mayo Clin Proc 2002; 77:429-436; Am J Med 2000;
109:95-101.

SUPERIOR VENA CAVA SYNDROME (SVC)

An itinerant dialysis patient

With stridor and swollen face, quite blatant.

Had past aortic dissection,

Brain blood made poor connection.

Ultrafiltration caused a marked improvement.

Note: This 44 year old homeless man traveled widely and irregularly dialyzed. On arrival he had a swollen face, over 20 lbs. of edema, loud respirations, and a median chest scar from an aortic dissection repair 5 years before. His upper airway was narrowed. Imaging showed obliterated jugulars and collaterals down his back. SVC was first described in 1757 by Hunter in a patient with a thoracic aortic aneurysm. Through the 1940's, case series were equally divided between chest cancers and aneurysms. Symptoms include face/neck/arm swelling, dyspnea, cough, chest pain, facial discoloration, and dysphagia. A current series of 78 patients had similar symptoms but a change in etiology. Neoplasia was seen in 60%, mainly lung cancer. However, 40% had non-malignant causes. Of these, 71% had intravascular devices as did 11% of the cancer patients. Only one had an aortic aneurysm.

Refs.: Medicine (Baltimore) 2006; 85:37-42; UpToDate.

EVERYTHING BUT EBOLA

Very ill woman came here from East Africa

With fever, malaise, and pancytopenia.

Lung infiltrates, was intubated;

And dialysis also indicated.

Her infections exceeded a trifecta.

Note: A 47 year-old Ethiopian woman was critically ill
at a local hospital with respiratory distress, oliguria,
and hypotension. There was also a right cerebral bleed
and lip blisters. She was ventilated, given pressors and
hemodialyzed. Lab tests showed: WBC - 0.3 K, platelets
- 22 K, CD4 – 11, and Hct – 22. A marrow aspirate
demonstrated toxoplasmosis. The lip lesions were due
to HSV-1. Pneumocystis was found in the lungs. A new
diagnosis of HIV was confirmed. All bacterial cultures
were negative. She survived on appropriate therapy.
Over one million Ethiopians have HIV, and there is
a sero-prevalence of 88% for Toxoplasma gondii in
them versus 50% in the general population. Positivity
correlates with eating raw meat and exposure to sheep
and goats.

Refs.: Epidemiol Infect 2012; 140:1935-1938; Infection
2013; 41:545-551.

ATRIAL FIBRILLATION IN ESRD

Warfarin treatment of Afib is common.

In fact, it's often a knee-jerk reaction.

Some recent studies have shown

Renal failure was bleeding-prone

Without patients gaining stroke protection.

Note: End-stage renal disease (ESRD) is accompanied by a subtle clotting problem (platelets don't aggregate well and many patients are on aspirin). Hemodialysis (HD) is conducted under heparin thrice weekly. I have observed serious bleeding complications in our hospital's ESRD/HD patients when some other provider started warfarin because of atrial fibrillation (Afib), as if it was a "magic bullet". However, amplifying the work of Hakim et al, a large Canadian study has introduced new evidence that warfarin was not beneficial in reducing stroke risk in dialysis patients with Afib and was associated with a 44% higher risk of hemorrhage. A randomized, multi-center, controlled trial is in order.

Refs.: Circulation 2014; 129:1196-1203; J Am Soc Nephrol 2009; 20:2223-2233.

OCCULT EMPHYSEMA

A large proportion of patients with "COPD"

Has no airflow obstruction on spirometry.

They still require smoking cessation,

May need different medication,

And our better defining etiology.

Note: "COPD exacerbation" is a major cause of emergency department visits and hospitalizations. COPD is defined as airflow obstruction that doesn't reverse. Most treatment of it targets the airways. Emphysema is characterized by destruction of intra-alveolar walls and can be diagnosed by chest CT scans. However, about half of COPD patients don't have much emphysema, but 10% of never smokers have it at autopsy. In a recent study of 2965 participants without airflow obstruction, aged 45-84 years receiving a cardiac CT scan, emphysema-like lung was associated with increased all-cause mortality, especially in smokers. A companion GWAS in never smokers showed links to genes highly relevant to alpha1-antitrypsin metabolism.

Refs.: Ann Intern Med 2014; 161:863-873; Am J Respir Crit Care Med 2014; 189:408-418.

FEBRILE TRANSPLANT PATIENT

Renal transplant patient, four months'
duration,

With fever, swollen neck, thigh aggravation.

CT showed abscesses galore,

Neck, thigh muscles and pelvic floor.

A Nocardia infection was the explanation.

Note: This man received induction immunosuppression
with methyprednisolone and alemtuzumab, followed
by prednisone, mycophenolate and tacrolimus
maintenance. Two months later watery diarrhea began
the illness. A 4.2 cm lung nodule was present. Aspirate
from one of the abscesses grew N. farcinica, which
represents 14% of CDC isolates of Nocardiae. It was
sensitive to Bactrim. Nocardiae are not part of human
flora. They are found world-wide in soil, decaying
vegetation, and water. Inhalation is the usual portal of
entry, but it can be directly inoculated; e.g. by an animal
scratch or bite. The patient owned dogs and cats. N. farcinica appears to be more virulent , is more likely to be
antibiotic-resistant, and to cause disseminated disease
than other Nocardiae. Because of a high recurrence rate,
6-12 months of therapy is needed.

Refs.: Eur J Clin Microbiol Infect Dis 2014; 33:689-702;
Clin Infect Dis 2007; 44: 1307-1314.

DOAN'S PILLS

CKD-5 with a very low bicarbonate,

Also not taking his sodium citrate,

Self-treating chronic back pain,

We looked up what it did contain,

Plenty of magnesium salicylate.

Note: This man was sent to Nashville from North Georgia without anyone taking a drug history. His serum creatinine was 5.9 mg/dl and his serum HCO3 was 8 meq/l. The serum anion gap was 25. There were no uremic symptoms. Although he had not been taking his prescribed sodium citrate due to its taste, this was not the whole answer. Most CKD-5 patients will have a HCO3 of 17-20 and an anion gap in the high teens without treatment. The "S" in increased anion gap metabolic acidosis acronyms (e.g. RED MULES) stands for salicylates. It is often forgotten. The number of over-the-counter remedies which contain various salicylates in the U.S. is staggering. Their toxicity is multi-systemic and can be confusing. Elderly patients in cold and flu season are significantly more at risk. This man was 82 years old.

Refs.: Arch Intern Med 1978; 138: 1481-1484; Seminars in Dialysis 1996; 9:257-264.

RUBEOLA IN AMERICA

School children are required to get this vaccination.

Many states make it easy to receive exemption.

Five Disneyland workers infected,

It spread to fifty unprotected.

"Powder keg needing a match" Schaffner's conclusion.

Note: The U.S. declared "red measles" eradicated in 2000, when only 86 cases were reported. This highly contagious viral pharyngitis is transmitted by coughing or sneezing on close contacts. In the intervening years less than 200 cases per annum were seen here. Most were linked to foreign travel or to foreign visitors. According to the CDC, 95% of U.S. schoolchildren have been vaccinated against rubeola. However, all states grant exemptions for medical reasons. All but 2 states extend this to religious objections. Nineteen states, including California, allow "philosophical differences" of parents to omit vaccination of their children. In certain areas this lowers the herd immunity to below the needed 92% or greater. Things changed in 2014; 644 cases of rubeola were reported to the CDC in 23 outbreaks. More than 80% were unvaccinated. The latest outbreak is ongoing.

Ref.: CDC website; BMC Public Health 2015; 15:447.

CRYPTOCOCCAL INFECTION IN ADVANCED AIDS

It causes meningoencephalitis severe,

Results in half a million deaths per year.

Make the call by antigen test.

Treat off ART is thought best.

After five weeks ART can reappear.

Note: Advanced AIDS is defined by very low CD4 counts. In sub-Saharan Africa the WHO recommends routine screening of AIDS patients with a CD4 count <100 cells/microliter for serum cryptococcal antigen (CrAg). In that region this fungus is the leading cause of adult meningitis. Early diagnosis and treatment lessens mortality. In a study of 87 such African patients, 39% had an abnormal neurologic exam and 48% had lost vision. Blindness was associated with high intracranial pressures. MRI brain scans detected cryptococcosis-related lesions in 63%. In the U.S., stored sera from 1986-2012 were examined in 1872 patients with advanced AIDS for CrAg. The prevalence was 2.9%. Positive patients had a shorter survival (2.8 years) than negative ones (3.8 years, P=.03). Recommendations for screening are the same as in Africa.

Refs.: J Infect 2014; Oct 22 (Loyse et al, Epub ahead of print); Clin Infect Dis 2014; Nov 24 (McKenney et al, Epub ahead of print).

B SYMPTOMS AT TWENTY EIGHT

Drenching sweats, weight loss, fever, SVC
syndrome,

Greatly enlarged anterior mediastinum,

To breathe he could not be supine.

Node biopsy the next thing in line.

Hodgkin's found, early therapy was
optimum.

Note: Over 9,000 patients are newly diagnosed with
Hodgkin lymphoma in the U.S. per year. Some familial
cases have occurred. There is an association with HIV or
EBV infection in a minority. Two peak incidences are in
young adults and in patients 55 years and older. More
than 80% present with lymphadenopathy above the
diaphragm, which involves the anterior mediastinum.
One third have B symptoms such as fever, night sweats,
and unintentional weight loss. Multiple node biopsies
may be needed to confirm the diagnosis because the
malignant Reed-Sternberg cells are scattered in a sea
of inflammatory cells. On a positive note, this is one of
the most curable neoplasms. Advances in radiation and
chemotherapy are leading to cures in 80% of Hodgkin
lymphoma patients younger than 60 years. Treatment
of relapses is discussed in the second paper. In this
patient, a course of glucocorticoids quickly alleviated his
symptoms.

Refs.: Mayo Clin Proc 2006; 81:419-426; Curr Hematol
Malig Rep 2014; 9:284-293.

RHEUMATOID   ARTHRITIS

Destructive joint inflammation hitting hard,

Prompt expert diagnosis is your hole card.

Other organs can be affected.

DMARDs are carefully selected.

Therapy is a battle with no holds barred.

Note: This autoimmune polyarthritis causes synovial
inflammation, leading to swelling, warmth, tenderness,
and stiffening. Female sex, genetics, and smoking
are risk factors. Small joints of the hands, feet, and
cervical spine are most commonly involved. It is
usually symmetrical. Knees and shoulders may be
injured too. Deformities result from tendon tethering
and erosion of joint surfaces. Disease-Modifying
Anti-Rheumatic Drugs (DMARDs) and biologics
are the primary treatment. In these categories are
methotrexate, leflunomide, TNF-alpha inhibitors,
interleukin-1 blockers, hydroxychloroquine, rituximab,
and, perhaps, glucocorticoids. NSAIDs don't alter the
natural history of RA. Early and aggressive treatment by
a rheumatologist, using at least one DMARD/biologic,
with close follow-up, yields the best results.

Refs: Arthritis Care Res (Hoboken) 2012; 64:625-639;
Ann Intern Med 2010; 153 (July 6):ITC1-ITC15.

COMPLICATIONS OF URINARY DIVERSION

High potassium and bicarbonate secretion,

Increased chemotherapy and antibiotic absorption,

Ammonia and oxalate excess,

Urine lytes and culture useless,

CKD from pyelo, reflux and obstruction.

Note: Ileal conduits and colonic neobladders have made the treatment of congenital GU tract problems and bladder cancer easier. Yet all of these patients develop complications (45% in 5 years and 100% in 15 years. Substances that have increased absorption are ammonia, lithium, sodium, chloride, oxalate, antibiotics and chemotherapeutic agents. A recent lymphoma patient here had two episodes of diffuse alveolar hemorrhage from his cecal bladder reabsorbing cyclophosphamide. Urinary wasting of K, HCO3, magnesium and calcium occurs. Resulting problems include osteomalacia, urinary infection, urolithiasis, gallstones, mental status changes, adenocarcinoma of the bowel segment, vitamin deficits, altered drug metabolism, multiple electrolyte changes, chronic renal disease, and acid-base disorders.

Refs.: Am J Med 1997; 102:477-484; J Urol 2003; 169:985-990.

RHABDO OF UNKNOWN ORIGIN (RUO)

Homeless man had fever and rhabdomyolysis.

Both legs were swollen, a compartment crisis?

No statin, ethanol, or cocaine,

Blood growing GPCs in a chain.

All explained by pneumococcal endocarditis.

Note: Rhabdomyolysis is often caused by prescribed medications, including their interaction. Chronic alcoholism, cocaine, trauma, arterial occlusion, compartment syndromes (CS), and others are on the list. Despite swollen tender legs, this man was not felt to have a CS by our surgeons. When Strep. pneumoniae grew from all 4 blood cultures, a PubMed search discovered 25 articles associating pneumococcal sepsis with rhabdomyolysis. A TTE next found an aortic valve vegetation. This organism can destroy a normal heart valve, and most often it is the aortic. Presumably, the leg findings were embolic. After an initial increase in the serum CK from 990 to 2900 in the hospital, penicillin G therapy returned the CK to normal. The patient had successful valve surgery.

Refs.: Weir, J R Soc Med 1998: 91:431-432; Hroncich, Am J Med 1989; 86:467-468; Bruyn, Q J Med 1990; 74 (273)33-40.

CAPNOCYTOPHAGA CANIMORSUS

Gram-negative rod escaping detection,

Frequently causes a fulminant infection.

Two-thirds have dog bites or licks.

Immunosuppressed are in a fix.

Occult sepsis, check for a canine connection.

Note: C. canimorsus was still unclassified in 1977 when 17 cases were reported. Its slow growth and requirement of a CO_2 atmosphere probably caused many patients to go undetected. The name of the genus means eater of CO_2. These are thin pleomorphic GNRs which can be seen in the gram stain of the buffy-coat of some patients. Asplenics are at particular risk of infection. This is a serious disease with multi-organ failure, DIC, and a 25% case fatality rate. In a study from Denmark, 26 of 39 patients were associated with being bitten or having a wound licked by a dog. An NEJM case would prick the blisters from his boots with an unsterile pin and let his dogs lick the wounds. Standard antibiotics are usually effective but there are no published trials that I know of.

Refs.: Pers, Clin Infect Dis 1996; 23:71-75; CPC, NEJM 1999; 340:1819-1826; Butler, Ann Intern Med 1977; 86:1-5; Alberio, NEJM 1998; 339:1827.

DIFFICULT TO CONTROL DIABETIC

Lowering his blood sugar I repeatedly tried,

But failure caused me to lose my pride.

Aetna blames me for the A1c,

But even they can clearly see

His tumor making glucagon on the slide.

Note: This thin man had a paradoxical combination of worsening diabetes and increasing insulin requirements, despite anorexia and weight loss. Our former Chief Resident, Charles Upchurch, who authored this limerick, discovered a locally invasive pancreatic neuro-endocrine tumor (PNET). At his request, a section of tumor stained strongly positive for glucagon. After a partial Whipple tumor resection, the patient's insulin needs decreased from 60-70 units to 10 units per day. In a series of 340 patients with PNETs only 7 per cent were glucagonomas. The glucagonoma syndrome includes a skin rash, diabetes mellitus, diarrhea, weight loss, DVTs, and neuropsychiatric symptoms. The neoplasms are firm encapsulated nodules from 2-25 cm in diameter. Many tumors are metastatic to liver (78%) at presentation. A number of treatments are available.

Refs.: Kindmark, Med Oncol 2007; 24:330-337; Bilimoria, Ann Surg 2008; 247:490-500; UpToDate.

A   GREAT   DISEASE

Untreated CLL admitted with neutropenia,

Months of dyspnea, sweats, worse asthenia.

PET scan positive on presentation;

Is this Richter's transformation?

Marrow showed granulomas and Histo fungemia.

Note: A "Great Disease" was coined locally by Dr. Roger Des Prez. It has at least three characteristics: lethality, esoteric presentations, and treatability (with possible cure). The more hopeless the initial situation is, the better the "eureka moment". It usually takes clinicians going the extra mile to solve the case, e.g. reviewing at length the sputum gram stain to find filamentous bacteria of Actinomyces, which were missed by routine laboratory tests. Pathologists love to find such patients for CPCs; e.g. a mitral stenosis patient with hemoptysis being treated for "vasculitis" with immunosuppression. Last week's glucagonoma of Dr. Upchurch was another example. The patient with CLL and histoplasmosis is now on itraconazole for a prolonged period as his cytopenias are being followed, and the possibility of an underlying lymphoma has not been dismissed.

Refs.: Luther, South Med J 2000; 93:692-697; Smith, Ann Intern Med 1972; 76:557-565.

HYPERCALCEMIA

It's common in patients with malignancy.

Eighty per cent is humoral from PTHrP

In cancers of lung, kidney and breast.

Osteolytic mets make up the rest.

Decreasing blood calcium eases symptoms quickly.

Note: The complexity of this topic increases as more molecular factors are implicated: PTHrP, RANKL, IL-1, IL-3, IL-6, IL-8, VEGF, MIP-1α, and calcitriol. Of non-skin neoplasms 20-30% are affected. Squamous cell carcinomas of lung/ head and neck, breast cancer, and multiple myeloma are the largest contributors. Non-specific symptoms and signs include nausea, vomiting, constipation, weight loss, mentation changes, and loss of renal function. Some patients present this way with undiagnosed neoplasms. It is important in these to make a diagnosis before proceeding. Almost all will need restoration of volume depletion. Loop diuretics aren't used because hypercalcemia acts like one. In the appropriate setting, inhibition of osteoclasts by drugs such as zoledronate is important in management.

Refs.: Mundy, J Am Soc Nephrol 2008; 19:672-675; Stewart, NEJM 2005; 352:373-379; Rosner, Clin J Am Soc Nephrol 2012; 7:1722-1729 (therapy).

THE EARLY 1980'S REVISITED

He had thrush, hypoxic respiratory failure,

Psych problems, wasting, known HIV exposure,

And cystic changes on chest x-ray.

Was bronchoscoped after some delay.

Pneumocystis the silver stain did capture.

Note: Before the recognition of HIV/AIDS, a prophetic article appeared on 6-5-81 in MMWR. Between 10-80 and 5-81, five young (29-36 years old) homosexual men were treated for Pneumocystis pneumonia in Los Angeles, CA. All of them had mucosal candidiasis (thrush) and current CMV infection. They did not know each other and had been previously healthy. The authors observed that this suggested " the possibility of a cellular-immune dysfunction related to a common exposure that predisposes individuals to opportunistic infections" (OIs). A month later MMWR reported the association of Kaposi's sarcoma and OIs in NY and CA in the gay population. Kaposi's is also an OI (HHV-8). This patient's lack of cooperation somewhat delayed his diagnosis. He is under treatment of his OIs. However, therapy of presumed HIV awaits a confirmatory test, which he is considering.

Refs.: MMWR 1981; 30:250-252; MMWR 1981; 30:305-308; Masur, NEJM 1981; 305:1431-1438.

URINARY   TRACT   LYMPHOMAS

Lymphoid cancer renal function devastates.

Diffuse large B-cell lymphoma predominates.

Masses, high calcium, obstruction,

Renal parenchymal infiltration,

And tumor lysis place kidneys in dire
straits.

 Note: I see several patients every year where lymphomas
of many types are complicated by renal insufficiency
or failure. Another facet of patient care is the plethora
of nephrotoxic medications which they are receiving.
Renal or GU sites represent less than 5% of primary
extranodal lymphomas. However, kidney biopsy has
revealed unsuspected B-cell lymphoma in 55 cases, eighty
per cent of which presented with AKI of unknown cause.
Nephrotic syndrome with intraglomerular involvement
was seen in 5 patients. Eighty per cent of the total had
interstitial lymphoma. Renal biopsy is also advocated as a
means of detecting angiotropic lymphoma. Treatment of
these disorders is based on the category of neoplasm.

Refs.: Mod Pathol 2009; 22:1057-1065; Am J Kidney Dis
2003; 42:960-971; Am J Med 1993; 94:133-139.

THE CENTOR SCORE IN PHARYNGITIS

One point each for lack of cough, having fever,

Anterior cervical nodes that are tender,

And tonsillar exudates,

Group A strep it separates.

Get strep antigen testing if two or greater.

Note: In adolescents and young adults, 80% of pharyngitis is viral with scores of 0 or 1. Group A streptococcus causes 10% and scores 2-4. These need to be quickly identified and treated with penicillin. Then there will be decreased symptoms, less contagion, and prevention of suppurative complications. A variety of organisms cause the other 10%. However, over 60% of U.S. patients receive antibiotics for sore throat. Many of these are contraindicated in group A strep, e.g. azithromycin and certain cephalosporins. Physicians should be aware that there are rare complicated cases of pharyngitis, such as Lemierre syndrome. In patients with a score of 3 or 4 and negative rapid tests for group A strep or lack of improvement in 24-36 hours of antibiotics, a broadened differential and further testing are in order.

Refs.: Ann Intern Med 2015; 162:241-247 and 311-312.

BACTERIAL SPINAL EPIDURAL ABSCESS

Most suffer with bad backache at admission.

Half have a prior vertebral condition.

Other diseases often preexist.

Rarity causes it to be missed.

Better imaging has led to faster recognition.

Note: Factors causing this problem to double in frequency in 20 years include an aging population, increasing chronic vascular access, more spinal instrumentation, and injection drug abuse. Bacteria gain entry through contiguous or hematogenous spread. About 70 per cent are infected with Staph aureus (half of these are MRSA). However, it is often difficult to pin down the initiating event causing bacteremia. This was true in a recent patient of mine with MSSA sepsis, who had large cervical and lumbar abscesses. Early treatment with decompressive laminectomy and appropriate antibiotics will lead to a better outcome. Hardware removal may be needed. Paralysis and death are seen when the diagnosis is delayed.

Refs.: Darouiche, NEJM 2006; 355:2012-2020; Maslen, Arch Intern Med 1992; 71: 1713-1721.

MANAGING GOUT

Treatment stopped due to flare, hard to figure out.

Tophi on all fingers, both heels extruded "grout".

The "grout" was withdrawn carefully,

Needle-shaped crystals on microscopy.

Diligence is needed to care for advanced gout.

Note: This disease has troubled mankind for millennia. It is due to a mutation in urate oxidase. Although very successful medications are now available to eliminate gout in compliant patients, there are many pitfalls in using them. Chief among these are patient non-compliance and physician errors in discontinuing drugs such as allopurinol or febuxostat because an attack of acute gouty arthritis occurred during therapy. The goal of treatment is to get the serum urate level under 6.0 mg/dl by blocking synthesis. A lower goal may be sought in patients with large sodium urate deposits (tophi) as here. Gouty flares should be treated with NSAIDs, colchicine or glucocorticoids, while continuing allopurinol or febuxostat. As the load of macro- and micro-crystalline sodium urate melts into the desaturated serum, the patient will be cured of gout (but the medication is needed life-long). The patient used the term "grout" for the texture of this crystalline heel exudate, likening it to the shower tile product.

Refs.: Ann Intern Med 2013; 158:906; Mayo Clin Proc 2006; 81:925-934; Nephrol Dial Transplant 2005; 20: 431-433.

THE TTKG AND POTASSIUM DISORDERS

If the source of low K is a mystery,

Calculate the test called the TTKG.

Measure K in plasma and urine

And osmolality in both to discern

Whether the kidneys are the main agency.

Note: This is a fractional excretion ratio which uses osmolality rather than creatinine in order to correct for water reabsorption in the medullary collecting tubule. However, the osmolality of the urine must be equal to or greater than the osmolality of plasma for the test to be valid. The equation is U/P potassium divided by U/P osmolality. In hypokalemia the response of normal kidneys is a TTKG of 1.0 or less. In hyperkalemia normal kidneys excrete K well with a TTKG of 8.0 or greater. Abnormal responses are the opposites. In hypokalemia fecal losses are the major other cause and are accompanied by low TTKGs (if the kidneys are normal). In a recent patient with hypokalemia which followed cisplatin treatment of cancer, the TTKG was 10, reflecting renal wasting. Low magnesium also plays a role there.

Ref.: Am J Kidney Dis 1994; 24:597-613.

RAPIDLY GROWING MYCOBACTERIA (RGM)

Environmental organisms that are found worldwide,

Isolated from soil, skin, fauna and everything beside.

Cause lung, bone, skin and soft tissue infection,

Spread further if there is immunosuppression.

Prolonged treatment a good result will provide.

Note: A beneficial aspect of these infections is that they can be be identified in a week, and their antimicrobial sensitivities determined. In this way they resemble typical bacteria. The major pathogens are M. abscessus, M. fortuitum, and M. chelonae. Pulmonary disease is predominantly due to the M. abscessus group (80%) and M. fortuitum (15%). M. chelonae often presents as a lymphocutaneous syndrome with complicating conditions including tattoo ink, pedicure water, joint prostheses, LASIK, and breast augmentations. A pedicure salon caused a mini-epidemic by nosocomial transmission of M. fortuitum. Once a patient is diagnosed with RGM infection, all foreign material must be removed . Drugs used for TB do not work. Empiric standard antimicrobials are effective in combination until sensitivity data return. Treatment may be needed for months. Infectious disease specialists should be involved. Experienced surgeons are sometimes needed.

Refs.: Griffith, Am J Respir Crit Care Med 2007; 175:367-416; NEJM 2002; 346:1366-1371.

FACTITIOUS LABORATORY MEASUREMENTS

If the lab test result does not make good sense,

It is high time for you to go on the offense.

Errors occur before analysis,

Such as in vitro hemolysis.

Hematologic conditions headline these events.

Note: There are mishaps before, during, and after blood test results are determined. Misinterpretation of hyperkalemia led to hemodialyzing a leukemic patient whose WBCs lysed during pneumatic tube transport, leading to release of K into serum. It was realized when hemodialysis did not correct the potassium. I made such a diagnosis in a child with Wilms tumor and a persistent serum K of 7.7 after 3 dialyses. This was due to thrombocytosis. The platelet count was 10 times normal, and they released lots of K in vitro during clotting in the test tube. The plasma K was normal. An EKG is also a good confirmation of the severity of hyperkalemia. Knowing that a serum phosphate of over 10 mg/dl does not happen when the serum creatinine is 3-4 mg/dl (unless exogenous phosphate is being taken) led to a diagnosis of occult multiple myeloma. This was due to paraprotein interference with the phosphate assay. One needs some handy references when confronted with the possibility of an artifact in a lab test.

Refs.: Am J Clin Pathol 2009; 131:195-204; Clin Chem 2002; 48:691-698.

ARACHNID   HEMOLYSIS

Brown recluse spider bites cause more than just pain.

Venom cleaves glycophorin from the red cell membrane.

It contains a sphingomyelinase,

Which activates metalloproteinase

Complement-mediated, could this Soliris restrain?

Note: The initially painless Loxosceles bite develops into an enlarging, painful necrotic lesion with surrounding erythema and ischemia. It also moves downhill in an elliptical shape. In some patients a severe intravascular hemolysis begins in the first 5 days. The HCT can decrease to half normal. Jaundice, hemoglobinuria, leukocytosis, thrombocytopenia, AKI, DIC and even death may occur. Small children are at particular risk. Treatment is supportive. The area should not be biopsied or debrided. Healing is slow over a period of weeks. Eculizumab (Soliris) is a monoclonal antibody targeting C5, which is used in the therapy of PNH and C3 glomerulopathies. It has been shown to be effective in vitro against Loxosceles reclusa venom-mediated hemolysis.

Refs.: Rosen, Ann Emerg Med 2012; 60:439-441; Gehrie PLoS One 2013; 8(9):e76558.

ZOONOSES FROM CATS

The biggest risks are cats not in a vet's care.

Agents include bites, claws, saliva, ticks they bear.

Infected fluids can aerosol.

Stool carries a pathogen haul.

Children and the immunosuppressed should beware.

Note: Feral cats are the worst. Although scratches and bites by the long, sharp teeth of any cat are emphasized (Bartonella henselae, Pasteurella multocida, Capnocytophaga), there are other dangers. Feline feces may carry Giardia, Toxocara cati, Toxoplasma gondii, Cryptosporidium, Campylobacter and other enteropathogens. Bordetella ("kennel cough") and Coxiella burnetii (birthing cats) can be aerosolized. Fleas and ticks on the cat may transmit ehrlichiosis, babesiosis, Yersinia pestis (plague), and tularemia to humans. Other rare transmissions are rabies, sporotrichosis, cowpox, leptospirosis, and tape worms. I want to underline that pregnant women are at great risk as well. Prevention is paramount. Regular veterinary care, control of fleas and ticks, feeding only high quality commercial cat food, claw clipping (by vet), and serious hand washing after litter box contact are standbys.

This subject is well covered in UpToDate. Also see Gerhold, Zoonoses Public Health 2013; 60:189-195.

LEAVE IT TO THE PROFESSIONALS

Never ascend a ladder with a chain saw.

A friend of mine broke this common sense law.

If you think you're saving money,

You are wrong, and it's not funny.

In abandoning this practice don't hem and haw.

Note: Like oil and water, these two items do not mix well. The recent incident involved a perfectly sane father of four scaling a ladder to trim some dead branches. After he fell (distance unknown), he may have arrived on the ground unconscious. This was presumably due to contact with the tree, ladder, or ground. It was unwitnessed. His wife found him like this with the chain saw still running nearby. He has completely recovered. A local medical faculty member was permanently injured in the same scenario. The damage to one arm resulted in the complex regional pain syndrome (CRPS), formerly known as reflex sympathetic dystrophy. He was in constant pain and could not function. Quality of life was seriously impaired. There also may be sensory, motor, and autonomic components of CRPS.

Ref.: Birklein, J Neurol 2005; 252:131-138.

Acute hyperammonemia's a bad situation;

Often is missed due to the patient's presentation.

Restless, tachypneic, combative,

Confused to quite unresponsive.

The outcome can be fatal brain herniation.

Note: The problems are that the underlying conditions are not usually linked to very high blood ammonia levels, the symptoms are non-specific, and it all happens acutely. I am not discussing undiagnosed urea cycle disorders, but they are in the differential. A report in 1988 found NHA in 8 leukemics and 1 lymphoma patient following chemotherapy. All but 1 died. In 2000, 6 of 145 orthotopic lung transplants developed NHA during the first 26 days post-grafting. Two-thirds died. In 2007 the pathophysiology and treatment of NHA in an ICU setting were discussed. When arterial ammonia levels are >200 mcmol/L, astrocytes rapidly metabolize it to glutamine. Osmotic effects of high intracellular glutamine lead to brain cell swelling and cerebral edema. Herniation ensues. Treatment is not always successful, partly due to delays in diagnosis.

Refs.: Am J Med 1988; 85: 662-667; Ann Intern Med 2000; 132:283-287; Chest 2007; 132:1368-1378.

New renal transplant still needing dialysis,

Poor urine output required analysis.

Wound opened, kidney was well perfused.

With biopsy they're no longer confused.

It showed the donor had rhabdomyolysis.

Note: Because of long renal transplantation waiting times due to lengthening lists of potential recipients, criteria for usable deceased donor organs have been "expanded" both in the U.S. and U.K. This refers to donors whose organs may be associated with worse outcomes. The crisis in supply compelled the transplant community to use as many of these kidneys as feasible. Another factor is that organs are obtained urgently and often shipped great distances. Clinical information may be incomplete. Autopsies aren't done on all donors. In a study from a major center, 85% of expanded donor kidneys were functioning at 3 years. This organ came from another state, and there was no mention of rhabdomyolysis in the note. Myoglobin casts were seen in the graft biopsy. However, this should be a recoverable state.

Refs.: Summers et al, Kidney Int 2015; Mar 18 (Epub ahead of print); Kosmoliaptsis et al, Am J Transplant 2015; 15:754-763.

PAINFUL   HEMATOCHEZIA

Man with diarrhea that was watery and
bloody,

Had rectal pain and recent cholecystectomy.

Proctoscopy showed an ulcer.

He lived with a male partner.

Chlamydia found in the ulcer on biopsy.

Note: Chlamydia trachomatis infection is the most
common notifiable infectious condition in the United
States. Almost all affected individuals are asymptomatic.
Over 1.4 million cases were reported to the CDC in 2011.
The CDC recommends annual screening of sexually
active women through 25 years old and for those over
25 with risk factors. PID is the worst complication.
All pregnant women should also be screened. (NAA
testing of vaginal swabs in women and first voided
urine in men). Heterosexual men who are in correctional
facilities, adolescent or STD clinics, or the military
should be screened as resources permit. It is also
recommended that men who have sex with men should
be screened annually at anatomical sites of exposure.
This man's partner was also Chlamydia positive. See first
reference about therapy.

Refs.: Ann Intern Med 2013; 158: ITC 2-1 to ITC 2-16
(Feb.5 issue); Workowski and Berman, MMWR; 2010; 59
(RR-12):1-110; UpToDate.

METABOLIC   MARVELS

During winter for six months bears
hibernate.

They don't move, eat, drink, defecate, or
urinate.

Using fat for energy,

Maintaining bone density,

There's complete reabsorption of renal
filtrate.

Note: Black and brown bears (Ursidae) hibernate in
underground dens and other sheltered spots to avoid
food deprivation. Their metabolism is reduced by
only 20-50%, and they arouse easily if awakened. Bears
have stored kilocalories as fat during hyperphagic
periods in autumn. While asleep in the den, their body
temperatures are 30-35 C, heart rates 8-10 BPM, and
oxygen consumption is half normal. Females can give
birth to cubs, lactate, and breast feed. BUN does not
increase. Ammonia is recycled into amino acids. Bone
stays normal without immobilization hypercalcemia.
Unlike humans, there are no pressure sores, blood clots
or pulmonary emboli. Muscle mass only decreases by
10-15%. Bears develop a proteolytic inhibitor which
blocks the muscle wasting of immobilization. They
awaken in the spring ready to go about their business.

Refs.: Stenvinkel, Kidney International 2013; 83:207-212;
Mayo Clin Proc 1987; 62:850-853.

IT'S NOT BUDD-CHIARI

Hematopoietic cell transplantation

May swiftly lead to sinusoidal obstruction,

Painful right upper quadrant,

Bilirubin increment,

And ten liter fluid accumulation.

Note: Hepatic sinusoidal obstruction syndrome (SOS) most often occurs in patients undergoing hematopoietic cell transplantation (HCT). It resembles Budd-Chiari, but the hepatic venous obstruction is due to occlusion of terminal hepatic venules and sinusoids rather than hepatic veins and IVC. SOS begins in the first 3 weeks of HCT with endothelial cell injury. Progressive venular occlusion leads to zonal liver disruption and hemorrhagic centrilobular necrosis, but the severity can be variable. Mean prevalence is 14%. Risk factors include high dose irradiation, cyclophosphamide, pre-existing liver disease, allogeneic grafts (vs. auto), young age and poor performance status. Fifty per cent develop acute kidney injury from hepatorenal syndrome and 25 % require hemodialysis.

Refs.: UpToDate; McDonald et al, 1993; 118:255-267.

THE APPROPRIATE URINARY CATHETER

Catheter-related infections we must deter.

A panel addressed three types of catheter

In every possible situation

With appropriate indication.

Ann Arbor rules will make our practice better.

Note: Beginning with the work of Kunin in the 1960's, the urinary catheter has been both a blessing and a curse. After reviewing the literature, a 15 member multidisciplinary team of physicians and nurses at the University of Michigan and its associated VA hospital has recently made recommendations about the use of Foley, intermittent straight, and condom catheters in 299 clinical scenarios of hospitalized medical patients. To refine criteria for appropriate catheter use (benefits outweigh risks), they applied the RAND/UCLA Appropriateness Method. Appropriate and inappropriate uses are covered for Foley (Table 2), intermittent straight (Table 3), and condom (Table 4) catheters. Table 5 summarizes the most common uses of each, with recommendations.

Refs. Meddings et al, Ann Intern Med (Supplement) 2015; 162:S1-S34; Kunin et al, NEJM 1966; 274:1155-1161.

PYODERMA GANGRENOSUM (PG)

A quickly developing purulent skin ulcer,

Painful, has a violaceous, undermined border.

Seen in inflammatory arthritis,

Crohn's disease and ulcerative colitis.

Avoid trauma, treat with an immunomodulator.

Note: PG is an uncommon inflammatory disorder which presents with skin ulcer(s). It is neither infectious nor gangrenous. Pathogenesis is uncertain. Differential diagnosis is broad. Half of PG patients have an underlying systemic illness. PG can be exacerbated at sites of trauma (pathergy). Severity of lesion(s) dictates therapy. There are no prospective randomized trials. Mild, localized disease may be treated with topical potent glucocorticoids or tacrolimus. Therapy of more extensive involvement requires systemic glucocorticoids and/or calcineurin inhibitors. Infliximab was effective in one trial. However, only half of PG patients achieve wound healing in one year. Almost all attain remission with longer follow-up. Relapses do occur.

Refs.: J Am Acad Dermatol 2005; 53:273-283; Medicine 2000; 79:37-46; UpToDate.

PAINFUL NODES AND UNUSUAL FEVER

Young man, who's a refugee from Somalia,

Has tender swelling in his left axilla.

He cuts up boxes in a factory,

Many sexual contacts by history,

And two times a day he has pyrexia.

Note: This 27 year-old African man had been in the U.S. since 2006. His last refugee camp was in Kenya. He was hospitalized here with a 4 day illness of malaise, fever, headache, and a sore, swollen axilla. He had cut his hand recently while dismantling boxes. The axilla was not fluctuant, erythematous or draining pus. A double quotidian fever was observed. Differential diagnosis of this includes visceral leishmaniasis, disseminated TB, GC endocarditis, typhoid fever, adult Still's disease, and a mixed malarial infection. Laboratory results revealed a CD4 count of 14, a positive HIV test, and Mycobacterium tuberculosis from the node. When there is newly discovered coinfection with TB and HIV, TB is treated first. If ART is begun early (1-4 weeks), TB-IRIS is twice as common, but survival is better when CD4 counts are under 50 cells/microL.

Ref.: Uthman et al, Ann Intern Med 2015; 163:32-39.

INDEX - VOLUME V

ABBREVIATIONS   VOLUME V

ADH	antidiuretic hormone
AFB	acid-fast bacillus
AIDS	acquired immunodeficiency syndrome
AKI	acute kidney injury
A1A	alpha1-antitrypsin
A1c	hemoglobin affected by diabetes
APAP	acetaminophen
ARB	angiotensin II receptor antagonist
ART	antiretroviral therapy
ATP	adenosine triphosphate
BAL	bronchoalveolar lavage
BK	nephropathic virus
BMT	bone marrow transplant
BP	blood pressure
BPM	beats per minute
BUN	blood urea nitrogen
CAA	cerebral amyloid angiopathy
CABG	coronary artery bypass graft
CaCO3	calcium carbonate
CAPD	chronic ambulatory peritoneal dialysis
CDC	Centers for Disease Control
CD4	type of lymphocyte
CK	creatine kinase
CKD	chronic kidney disease
Cl	chloride
CLL	chronic lymphocytic leukemia
CMV	cytomegalovirus
CNI	calcineurin inhibitor

CNS	central nervous system
COPD	chronic obstructive pulmonary disease
CO2	carbon dioxide
COX-2	cyclooxygenase-2
CPC	clinicopathologic conference
CRPS	complex regional pain syndrome
CS	compartment syndrome
CSF	cerebrospinal fluid
CT	computed tomography
C3 or C5	complement component
CYP3A4	cytochrome p450 3A4
DFA	direct fluorescent antibody test
DIC	disseminated intravascular coagulation
DIL	drug-induced lupus
DKA	diabetic ketoacidosis
DMARDs	disease-modifying anti-rheumatic drugs
DNA	desoxyribonucleic acid
DVT	deep venous thrombosis
EBV	Epstein-Barr virus
ED	emergency department
EGD	esophagogastroduodenoscopy
EGFR	epidermal growth factor receptor
EKG	electrocardiogram
ERCP	endoscopic retrograde cholangio-pancreatography
ESRD	end-stage renal disease
FDA	Food and Drug Administration
GC	gonococcal, gonococci
GFR	glomerular filtration rate

GI	gastrointestinal
GNR	gram-negative rod
GPA	granulomatous polyangiitis
GPC	gram-positive coccus
GU	genitourinary
HAART	highly active antiretroviral therapy
HCO3	bicarbonate
HCT	hematocrit or hematopoietic cell transplant
HCTZ	hydrochlorthiazide
HCV	hepatitis C
HD	hemodialysis
HER2	an oncogene
HHV	human herpes virus
histo	histoplasmosis
HIV	human immunodeficiency virus
HOCM	hypertrophic cardiomyopathy
HPV	human papillomavirus
HSV	Herpes simplex virus
IBD	inflammatory bowel disease
ICU	intensive care unit
IgE	immunoglobulin E
IgM	immunoglobulin M
IL	interleukin
IMA	inferior mesenteric artery
IRIS	immune reconstitution inflammatory syndrome
IV	intravenous
IVC	inferior vena cava
IVIG	intravenous immunoglobulin
K	potassium

KCNJ11	gene for a potassium channel
LASIK	laser-assisted surgery on the cornea
LC	immunoglobulin light chain
LP	lumbar puncture for spinal fluid
LVAD	left ventricular assist device
MAC	Mycobacterium avium complex
MCA	middle cerebral artery
MEN	multiple endocrine neoplasia
MERS	Middle East respiratory syndrome
MFS	Marfan syndrome
MGUS	monoclonal gammopathy of uncertain significance
MIP	macrophage inflammatory protein
MPXV	monkeypox virus
MRI	magnetic resonance imaging
MRSA	methicillin-resistant Staphylococcus aureus
MSSA	methicillin-sensitive Staphylococcus aureus
mTOR	mammalian target of rapamycin
Na	sodium
NAA	nucleic acid amplification
NF	neurofibromatosis
NFKB	nuclear factor kappa beta
NHA	non-hepatic hyperammonemia
NMS	neuroleptic malignant syndrome
NSAID	nonsteroidal anti-inflammatory drug
OI	opportunistic infection
osm	osmolality

OTC	over the counter (non-prescription)
PCP	primary care provider
PCR	polymerase chain reaction
PD	peritoneal dialysis
PDB	Paget's disease of bone
PE	pericardial effusion
PET	positron emission tomography
P53	a tumor suppressor gene
PG	pyoderma gangrenosum
PID	pelvic inflammatory disease
PNET	pancreatic neuroendocrine tumor
PNH	paroxysmal nocturnal hemoglobinuria
PR	segment of the EKG
psych	psychiatric
PTHrp	parathyroid hormone-related peptide
PTSD	post-traumatic stress disorder
RA	rheumatoid arthritis
RANK	receptor activator for NFKB
RANKL	ligand for RANK
RBC	red blood cell
RGM	rapidly growing mycobacteria
RHS	Ramsay Hunt syndrome
RMSF	Rocky Mountain spotted fever
RSV	respiratory syncytial virus
RUO	rhabdomyolysis of unknown origin
SAP	serum alkaline phosphatase
SBE	subacute bacterial endocarditis
SIADH	syndrome of inappropriate ADH
SMA	superior mesenteric artery

SOS	hepatic sinusoidal obstruction syndrome
ST	segment of the EKG
STD	sexually-transmitted disease
SVC	superior vena cava
SVT	supraventricular tachycardia
TB	tuberculosis
T4	thyroxine
TGF	transforming growth factor
TKR	total knee replacement
TNF	tumor necrosis factor
TSH	thyroid stimulating hormone
TTE	transthoracic echocardiogram
TTKG	transtubular potassium gradient
ULN	upper limit of normal
U/P	urine to plasma ratio
URI	upper respiratory infection
UT	University of Texas
UV	ultraviolet
VA	Veterans Affairs
VEGF	vascular endothelial growth factor
VU	Vanderbilt University
WBC	white blood cell
WHO	World Health Organization
WNV	West Nile virus

Made in the USA
Las Vegas, NV
09 February 2022

43565329R00066